DR. LEWIS JASSEY

I dedicate this book to my grandfather, David, for inspiring me to work with children. And you weren't even a pediatrician. You fixed belts for a living. But when I was very young, you taught me a trick. You showed me how to make a child smile. You could do it at will. Even when a child was crying hysterically. I still try to be just like you, every day.

And to my grandmother, Eva, and my mother, Carla. You both taught me how to bring the written and spoken word to life. I also want to thank my mom for keeping me disciplined and focused on my education. There were many times you wouldn't let me go to the park to play football with my friends until I finished my homework, and when I was livid you told me someday I'd understand and thank you for it. Well, I truly do. I wouldn't be where I am today without you.

And to my father, the late Dr. Marvin Jassey, whom I miss terribly, I want to thank you for two things. Number one, for bringing me with you on those house calls, even when no one else was doing house calls anymore. Patients often referred to you as an extension of their family, and that was a lure that pulled me toward medicine. And in your inspirational fight for your life against Lou Gehrig's disease, you taught me a very valuable lesson in courage and tenacity, and refusing to give up in what you believe in. I still feel that a part of you is with me every day.

DR. JONATHAN JASSEY

I dedicate this book to our late father, Dr. Marvin Jassey. I remember in first grade, I had a show-and-tell, and my father came to class to show X-rays and talk about being a doctor. I can honestly say from that instant, I knew I wanted to be just like him. This was something

I was destined to become and I have him to thank for inspiring me. I have already done the same thing for my two oldest daughters' classes and they seem to be as inspired as I was at that age.

I also want to dedicate this book to all the patients and parents at Bellmore Merrick Pediatrics and Adolescent Medicine who trusted in the Jassey Way. Some of you laughed and thought, "No way this can happen." But you put your faith in us and we got you to that promised land. Thanks for believing in us. And to those people out there who don't think something like this is possible because no one has ever shared this information with them—it is possible.

CONTENTS

Well Baby Exams

Newborn · 1 Month · 2 Months · 3 Months · 4 Months · 5 Months · 6 Months · 9 Months · 1 Year · 15 Months · 18 Months · 2 Years

Let There Be Sleep!

Why Sleep Train?

As pediatricians with more than thirty years of combined experience, we've helped countless parents sleep train their newborns, with great success—regardless of whether they were first-time parents, skeptical about the process or eagerly on board from the start. To address the desires and concerns of parents who approach sleep training from different angles, we've written a few letters to them (feel free to read them all or just the one that best applies to you and your family).

Letter to the First-Time Mom

Hi First-Time Mom!
Congratulations on the new addition to your family and welcome to the most exciting, amusing, difficult, mystifying and downright rewarding adventure you could ever hope to have on this earth.

One of the first questions we ask new moms and dads we see in our practice is: "Do you want your baby to sleep through the night?"

Since you're reading this book, your answer is probably "Yes," or at least "Maybe . . . as long as it's safe" or something similar. Or perhaps it's "Yes! Good Lord, yes!" Those are the most common reactions we get.

But some parents look at us like it's a trick question. Like they're thinking:

"This is a test. Infants aren't supposed to sleep through the night, they need to be fed constantly, like a parking meter, and if we act like we don't know that, Dr. Jassey is going to report us to child services."

Well, it's not a trick question. It's not a test. It's more a politely rhetorical question, a transition question from which we can flow into our signature spiel, where we explain our sleep training method, "the Jassey Way."

The reason that this question is not totally rhetorical is that some parents actually answer "No!"

We rarely see them, but some parents do think that having a baby that doesn't sleep through the night, and being miserably tired all the time as a result, is sometimes just an inevitable part of parenting. And that that's all there is to it.

But the truth is, we want all parents to answer our question with a "Yes. Yes, I want my baby to sleep through the night." And there's a simple reason for that.

Our job is to look after the well-being of the child, and in that capacity, we're responsible for giving parents all of the tools they need to promote and protect that child's well-being. And one of the most important tools parents can have is being well rested themselves. Being well rested helps parents to be not only more alert, but happier. It makes them better parents.

That's the one-line argument for sleep training, new mom:

A happier, more alert parent is a better parent.

So we'd prefer that your newborn not keep you up all night. Because the only way you can consistently get the good night's sleep you need to be the best parent you can be is for your baby to get a good night's sleep, too.

So please—let there be sleep!

Sincerely,

Lewis and Jonathan Jassey

Letter to the Experienced Mom

Hi Experienced Mom,

If your previous child (or children) did not sleep through the night, and left you tired and possibly unhappy much of the time as a result, then we probably don't have to convince you of the merits of sleep training. The concept sells itself!

But if your previous child was one of the rare, miracle babies that slept through the night almost automatically, then there's probably not much we could say to convince you that this next child will be any different. You're probably going to want to ride that hot streak. We're realists. We know how it is. We've seen it all before.

But we do beseech you to keep this book handy, because we assure you: Siblings rarely take after each other in their ability to sleep through the night without training. And there may soon come a time when you rise up and finally exclaim: "Let there be sleep!"

Be warned!

Sincerely,

Lewis and Jonathan Jassey

Letter to the Mom Who Thinks Sleep Training May Be Harmful

Dear Mom Who Would Consider Sleep Training, But Thinks It May Be Harmful to Her Baby,
We understand your concern, because there's a lot of misinformation out there. Some so-called experts theorize that babies aren't "meant" to sleep overnight, period; that they need to be fed on a twenty-four-hour cycle. Others will tell you that babies can only be sleep trained at a certain age, and that it's asking too much of them physically and mentally before then.

These claims are just not true. They might be completely well intentioned, but they're also unfounded.

As we'll address in more detail in the following pages, there is no established evidence that infants need to feed overnight to maintain healthy weight gain or development, or that being trained to sleep overnight puts at risk a baby's long-term health.

In reality, the arguments against baby sleep training are emotional, not rational.

Have you ever had a friend who's afraid of flying? You show them all the irrefutable statistics proving that air travel is the safest mode of transportation available, but while they're happy to get in a car, going up in the sky in a jet remains out of the question. Even they admit their fear is not rational; it's purely emotional.

We can look at baby sleep training in much the same way. All objective evidence points to it being safe.

So please, do yourself—and your child—a favor. Let there be sleep!

Sincerely,
Lewis and Jonathan Jassey

Why Choose This Book?

You can't eat sushi. You can't smoke. You can't smoke marijuana. You can't smoke crack. You can't jump on trampolines. It's basically a giant list of things you can't do.

—Father-to-be Seth Rogen, describing a baby book to mother-to-be Katherine Heigl, in *Knocked Up*

A Brief History of Baby Care

Did you know that human beings have been having babies for about two hundred thousand years? It's true; for as long as people, in our present biological form, have existed, we've been having babies. And since we, as a species, began speaking languages only around a hundred thousand years ago, that means that we were having babies for around a hundred thousand years before any caveman or -woman could even have *dreamed* of composing a *baby book*.

But you wouldn't know it from reading these books today. Too many baby care books, baby sleep books included, tend to treat infants as if they're delicate Fabergé eggs balancing on slanted rooftops; if Mommy or Daddy even *look* in the wrong direction, baby will come tumbling down and shatter to pieces. The way these books tell it, the fact that the human race has reproduced, let alone *prospered* as long as it has is nothing short of a miracle.

Okay, we exaggerate. But we agree with Seth Rogen's character in the 2007 movie *Knocked Up*—because *someone* has to lighten the mood here in the Land of Baby Care Literature. That's also why we had the Eagles classic "Take It Easy" in our heads while writing much of this book. Because the happy truth is that your baby is a supremely resilient little creature. You think your MacBook Air can take a good licking? You think a Bugaboo stroller is an indomitable fortress? These things are impressive, but could they have survived during, say, the Stone Age?

Babies did.

Babies.

. . .

Needless to say, not *all* babies survived such periods, and tragically, even in this day and age, there are babies all over the world suffering from want.

But if you bought this book, or if someone gave it to you, the odds are overwhelming that you possess the fundamental physical and emotional resources required to raise a perfectly healthy baby—with the help of a relatively small amount of important advice.

Most experienced parents (moms and dads who have had a child before) know this already, of course. They've learned it from the best possible baby guide there is: a living, breathing, growing baby. They tend to be much more confident with the second baby. But it's not just that they've acquired a whole set of parenting skills from the first child. It's also the case that they've learned they don't have to be so afraid of screwing up, as Jessica S., whose daughters are our patients, put it:

> *You're much more cautious with everything [the first time]. You're sterilizing the pacifier every time it hits the floor. Now you're rinsing it off. You realize babies aren't as delicate as you'd think.*

But too many parents don't seem to understand this. They fear that if they're not keeping up with the latest books and theories on parenting, and applying them to their children immediately, they're negligent somehow. They're not.

So we want to make that point up front, because if we're about to give you more than a hundred pages of parenting "advice," we want to make sure that you understand that, should you not follow our advice, it would not imply that you are a "bad" parent. Because chances are, as long as you are a thoughtful parent with positive intentions, your child is going to be just fine.

And we don't only say that to ease your mind. We say it because more than anything else—well, besides your child being healthy—we want you to *enjoy* this time. We're not sure that we're eloquent enough to properly capture in words the magic of parenthood, but let's just say that it's not something you want to miss out on, if you can at all help it.

But scared parenting is like scared driving; it doesn't accomplish its own aim, and it removes any joy you get from the activity in the process. We want you to have confidence! As we said, if you're reading this book, chances are you totally have what it takes to raise a great kid.

Navigating the Rough Waters of Baby Sleep Advice

If you go on any Internet message board or blog, you'll see endorsements for any number of sleep training methods, many of them completely at odds with one another. And yet moms swear by them just the same.

We are confident that the Jassey Way is the best baby sleep training method. We are confident it offers moms and dads the best chance to get their children sleeping through the night. Our ballpark estimate is that, since we started coaching parents in the Jassey Way in our practice over fifteen years ago, nine out of ten parents who have followed through on it have been successful.

But you've no doubt heard of the success of other methods, and you've seen Internet message boards that endorsed various strategies, and you surely have friends who have sworn by other baby sleep books. So it might be helpful to explain why, when you get right down to it, *all* baby sleep books and methods are pretty similar and are all fairly successful.

The reason for this assertion is pretty simple: All baby sleep books have two *extra* guarantees built into them.

The first: *All babies sleep, and some babies naturally sleep through the night on their own.*

Certainly, only *some* babies come equipped with this skill on their own, not *most* or even *many*; but we do see it.

So your baby might sleep through the night *no matter which book you read*—or even if you don't read any book at all. In fact, you could be completely illiterate, and your baby might sleep like a rock from day one.

All this is to say that *every* baby sleep book has a fighting chance of succeeding, no matter what procedures it advocates.

The second baby sleep book guarantee: *The core of any baby sleep training method is routine.*

Babies are creatures of habit. And they depend on environmental cues to know what to do and when. So getting your baby to sleep through the night is largely a matter of *conditioning* her to do so. It's a matter of building a framework of routine around your baby's daily life that enables a long nighttime stretch during which she is accustomed to sleeping.

Whether it's putting your baby to bed at a particular time

every night, always reading or singing to your baby to help her to sleep, making sure lighting and other environmental factors remain constant, sticking to a consistent feeding schedule, or whatever else, you'd be hard-pressed to find a baby sleep training method that didn't have some kind of *routine* at the heart of it.

When we combine these two certainties—that some babies will sleep through the night on their own, and that getting any baby used to a daily routine increases the chances that that baby will sleep through the night—we can see why *any* baby sleep book or method has at least a decent chance of success.

And since this is such a personal issue for moms and dads, it's easy to understand how, if one method works for a particular family, they might come to trumpet that method and critique others—even if they have no personal experience with them.

Now that we've explained how we're not special, let's talk about how we are.

WE KEEP IT REAL

We don't mean to brag, but: We never intended to write a book about baby sleep. We are in this to help babies and parents. When it comes to baby sleep, we 100 percent keep it real.

Our sleep training method, the Jassey Way, was something we would simply explain to the parents we saw in our pediatric practice. We'd ask, "Do you want your baby to sleep through the night?" and if the answer was "Yes," we would explain our method. We were happy when the parents reported back to us that it was successful, but our baby sleep ambitions never extended beyond the walls of our office in Bellmore, Long Island.

But over the years, more and more parents we saw in our

practice started telling us, "You have to write a book about it," in reference to our sleep method. Eventually, enough of them said it that we decided to do it.

So you see, the Jassey Way wasn't developed from studies, or lab tests, and it hasn't been "proven" by them, either. It comes from the sum total of treating more than fifteen thousand babies over the course of more than thirty years combined of practicing pediatrics.

The bottom line: The Jassey Way has worked for the families we treat. It's worked for enough of them that we can say, with confidence, that it should work for *most* babies; it's more a matter of whether or not you want to *use* our method, than of whether or not it will work.

THE PROCESS IS STRAIGHTFORWARD

Some baby sleep books read more like incredibly detailed manuals for do-it-yourself furniture or electronics assembly.

We're talking about the books that advocate Olympic figure skating–like routines surrounding the nightly act of putting the child to bed: meticulous, time-consuming multistep procedures involving highly calibrated lighting, scripted spoken lines, check-ins at various intervals, keeping sleeping logs—those sorts of things. We're talking about sleep training methods that might succeed by making you a MD/PhD in baby sleep, when all you need is a little undergrad-level summer course.

In contrast, the Jassey Way is very structured, sure, but it is not at all complicated, complex, or particularly demanding of your time.

WE'RE ALL ABOUT COULD, NOT SHOULD

Some baby sleep books—not to mention baby care books as a whole—take a "my way or the highway" approach to sleep training. Their theories might be sound, and their methods generally effective, but they are so rigid in their recommendations that they may give the reader the impression that if he or she doesn't do exactly as they say, that if the reader doesn't stay 100 percent on their course, that the reader is being somehow negligent. These books run the risk of leaving readers more afraid of what they *shouldn't* be doing with their child than what they *could* be doing.

Call us old-fashioned, but we think raising a baby should be a joyous, life-affirming experience for moms and dads. It should be a time marked by overwhelming love and the making of warm, long-lasting memories. It should be a time of reliving the wonders of early life through your baby's eyes. It should not be a time shadowed by an ever-present black hole of worry—a constant fear of doing something wrong—that can swallow so much of the joy of being a new parent.

So this book is *not* about the things you *shouldn't* be doing while raising your baby. Of course, we'll cover some of those things—we'd be negligent not to. But our focus is on *doing* the one thing that, more than anything else, in our thirty-plus years of practicing pediatrics, frees parents from the exhaustion and anxiety that too often stands between them and the pure joy of raising a baby.

Remember the old NyQuil commercials that told us that the medication was more than a simple cough syrup? That it was "the nighttime, sniffling, sneezing, coughing, aching, stuffy head, fever so you can rest medicine"?

Think of the Jassey Way as "the day and nighttime baby feeding, soothing, and sleeping so you can have the energy and confidence to truly enjoy the magic of early parenting without pulling your hair out sleep training."

BUT THIS BOOK WON'T PUT YOU TO SLEEP

All homages to NyQuil notwithstanding, at the risk of sacrificing any perceived modesty on our part, we'd be remiss not to say that we're fun guys. When you treat kids all day, you *have* to be entertaining; it's the only way to really get their attention.

And let's be honest: Are adults really so different?

We want this book to *work* for you, but if you don't enjoy reading it, you're less likely to pay attention to what we say in it in the first place. So we tried to make all of this less clinical and more lighthearted and fun.

(Emphasis on *tried*.)

How to Read/Use This Book

YOU DON'T HAVE TO GO IN ORDER

You have a newborn who may or may not be keeping you up at night, you have a family, you have a job, you're juggling a thousand responsibilities and obligations every day; you don't have the time, energy or, frankly, interest necessary to dive into this book like it's the Old Testament and you're a biblical scholar.

You need to be able to get valuable information out of this book even if the best you can do is pick it up at random moments and possibly read it out of order.

For those reasons, we've structured this book so that you can, for the most part, read any chapter on its own. Unavoidably, some chapters contain references to previous chapters, but none of these will "trip you up" if you haven't already read the chapter in question.

Ideally, you'll read this book in order, but by no means do you have to for it to be effective.

THE PARENTS' BILL OF RIGHTS

At the beginning of Chapters 2, 3, 4 and 5, you'll immediately see a section called the Parents' Bill of Rights. Each of these chapters presents an "article" of the bill, which highlights some of the most important points we'd like to make about that particular aspect of baby care—and which will hopefully give you the kind of no-nonsense, global perspective on that subject that's necessary for healthy parenting. These subjects include sleep training, crying, sleeping yourself, and breast and bottle feeding.

We included this Bill of Rights because, in our experience, too many parents simply don't *know* their "rights." They've been inundated with so many myths and falsehoods, and so much inaccurate "wisdom" has been passed down to them, that we wouldn't miss an opportunity to set the record straight—in bold type.

We hope that this Bill of Rights will serve as a comfort to parents during the moments of doubt that these topics often produce.

"JUST GIVE ME THE SLEEP TRAINING, PLEASE."

If you'd like to cut straight to learning our sleep training method itself, and you aren't very interested in any additional baby care enrichment, you can get by reading *only* Chapter 2, "The Jassey Way (Eat Right, Sleep Tight)."

That will take you through our method, step-by-step, in its entirety.

A Note on Language

In a book like this, it's impossible to avoid using gender-specific pronouns on a frequent basis. For the sake of simplicity and consistency, we exclusively use female pronouns when referring to your baby. For example, take the following sentence: "If your baby learns to sleep through the night, SHE will be better able to self-soothe later on in life." That statement applies to both male and female children, not just females.

Similarly, we often refer to *your* baby and babies in general (*all* babies, so to speak) interchangeably.

Unless otherwise noted, any statement we make about any baby refers to *your* baby as well, male or female.

The Newborn Sleep Problem

Lewis remembers the first time he was inspired to share our baby sleep method with a patient. He had just done a routine one-month newborn checkup on a little girl named Juliana.

While baby Juliana seemed perfectly well, first-time mother Jessica appeared frazzled and unhealthy. The bags under her eyes were substantial, her hair was disheveled, and she had a slight quiver in her voice as if ready to cry any moment.

"I'm falling apart," Jessica said. "I barely sleep three hours a night. I don't shower every day anymore. I can't think straight. I'm a physical and emotional wreck."

Then her husband, Paul, chimed in.

"I get more sleep taking catnaps at the office than I do at home," he said.

"One time I fell asleep in the rocking chair while breast-feeding," Jessica said. "I woke up as she was slipping through my arms. It was frightening."

She went on to recount all the old-fashioned tricks and advice her parents and friends recommended to get the baby to sleep through the night, none of which worked. Cooled chamomile tea, gripe water, water from boiled rice—nothing worked. Heck, she even pulled a small pint bottle of whiskey out of her purse.

"Doc, just gimme the word," she said. "I'll put it in her bottle."

Lewis looked into her bloodshot eyes and sensed her feelings of helplessness and despair. At that point, he knew he was facing an opportunity to make a real difference. In the life not only of a newborn, but of an entire family.

Lewis went on to tell Jessica and Paul about a method we had been developing for getting a baby to sleep soundly through the night—one that was based on a wealth of experience and simple common sense.

That's what this book is about: Getting your newborn to sleep through the night. Plain and simple. Specifically, we're talking about at least seven hours of uninterrupted, whiskey-free sleep.

We've been practicing pediatrics for thirty years combined, during which time we've cared for more than fifteen thousand newborns. We have second-generation patients—children of children we've treated. We live and breathe and love our jobs.

We've continually researched and practiced our method, adjusted, and practiced some more. We consulted with leading pediatric gastroenterologists. We listened to our patients as they provided feedback on what worked and what didn't, who demonstrated faith in our method and helped refine it over time, until we finally felt comfortable calling it "the Jassey Way."

We've also been on the other side of the stethoscope, as it were; as new parents, we've had that "deer in headlights" feeling—despite being board certified pediatricians.

We always have that empathy when our patients walk into the examination room. We understand how parenting hastens countless questions, issues, and concerns that few of our prior life experiences have prepared us for. We understand that people cling to a doctor's words, for better or for worse. We understand that we have to be careful how we guide people; we take that to heart.

So we absolutely mean it when we say that seven hours of uninterrupted sleep is an exceedingly achievable goal for a newborn. It is not only exceedingly achievable; it is exceedingly beneficial, for baby and parents alike.

The baby sleep problem is nothing new; sleepless nights for newborns and, by extension, their parents and siblings, constitute an issue as old as parenting itself. We've all come to think of sleepless nights as a rite of passage for new parents, as inevitable as changing diapers.

Whether you are reading these pages before or after your baby's arrival, your friends and family have undoubtedly bombarded you with countless questions and remarks about sleep. "Are you getting any sleep?" "Get all the sleep you can now. You won't get any once the baby arrives." "Is the baby a good sleeper?"

Before you're a parent yourself, the idea of getting no sleep in the service of taking care of your new baby sounds annoying and maybe even torturous, but it also sounds heroic and adventurous. It's literally the stuff of sitcom television; from 2011 to 2012, NBC ran a show called *Up All Night*, starring Christina Applegate and Will Arnett as new, sleepless parents.

It all seems so normal—so inevitable—that when we ask new parents our usual question—"Do you want your baby to sleep through the night?"—many of them think it's a trick question. They look confused, afraid to say yes even though every fiber of their being is screaming "For the love of God, yes!"

Not only is this not a trick question, but it's a very necessary question, as a sleepless baby can have a harmful trickle-down effect on the whole family. A sleepless infant might have trouble self-soothing later on in life—might be a less well-adjusted person. These conditions aren't inevitable either, but they're a very real concern.

We know this well because our philosophy of pediatrics is that it's a discipline with three dimensions: the current health and well-being of the child; the health and well-being of the adult that that child will grow up to be; and the health and well-being of the immediate family members that will influence and be influenced by that child.

We learned this as young children ourselves, as we accompanied our father, Dr. Marvin Jassey, on house calls—intimate experiences that impacted how we see the patient not as a stand-alone individual, but rather as part of a larger family system, simultaneously influencing and being influenced by others in the home.

Each member of the family has his or her own set of feelings, emotions, needs, wants, and capabilities, all of which are in flux, especially following the arrival of a new baby. Mommy, Daddy, big brother and/or sister, perhaps even the family pet, are all affected. We have always viewed our duty not only as treating our newborn patient, but also as helping the entire family enjoy a smooth transition and peaceful environment, one where baby's arrival does not necessarily upend the home's harmony and routine. Understanding the family situation and "treating the family" requires a fair amount of two-way dialogue between the patient and the doctor. It's the reason we allot thirty minutes for each well visit/checkup, when the industry norm is only ten, and sometimes fewer.

And so it is with the health and well-being of the entire family in mind that we developed the Jassey Way, a proven method to get your newborn sleeping at least seven consecutive hours through the night by the time she celebrates her one-month birthday.

Truth be told, most who begin sleep training as soon as they return home from the hospital, which is preferable, accomplish this goal in half that time. By the time your child lifts his or her own head or coos at the sound of your voice, your little bundle of joy will also be sleeping through the night. More importantly, so will you!

Sleep Training and Self-Soothing

One side benefit of the Jassey Way is that in addition to synchronizing the baby's sleep schedule with that of the rest of the Western world, as we alluded to earlier, it provides early opportunities for your baby to self-soothe. Self-soothing is one of the earliest and most important independence milestones that a baby must reach, not only because it makes life far more pleasant for the family, but also because children who never learn to self-soothe tend to struggle with future milestones of independence, such as sleeping alone, potty training, parental separation, and beyond.

Then, before you know what happened, that child is reaching a milestone you never anticipated: being cast on Bravo!'s *Princesses: Long Island*.

Bottom line: Self-soothing is an important life skill.

THE JASSEY WAY

At the core of our method is the undeniable direct relationship between eating—specifically, digesting—and sleeping. The Jassey Way calls for managing the baby's eating schedule so that all nutrients and calories are provided during "normal business hours" rather than the well-intended—but misguided—twenty-four-hour drive-thru schedule that most parents come to find unsustainable, exhausting, and ultimately unhealthy. The Jassey Way takes advantage of not only how digestion affects sleep, but also how daytime schedules and nighttime schedules act upon each other. To put it another way: It not only makes nighttime better, but it makes daytime better, too.

One question we're often asked is "Will the Jassey Way involve listening to a lot of crying at night?" The short answer is that it's entirely up to you.

Babies cry, sleep training or not, and if you are around to hear it, we know that it can be unsettling, particularly if you're left guessing at the cause.

That's why we devote an entire chapter to crying (Chapter 3, "The Crying Game"). We discuss in detail why babies cry, why you have an emotional and visceral reaction to it, and what to do about it—if anything.

The real issue with crying at night is how long it's going to be an issue. Essentially, you have the option of enduring a few weeks of it—as you show baby the way of the world—or one to two years or more of it.

Consider this: According to a 2010 study published by the National Institute of Health (NIH), roughly 50 percent of "typically developing infants" sleep for eight hours at a stretch at five months of age.[1]

This begs the question "When do the other 50 percent of families finally get a good night's sleep?"

The answer is that it varies, of course, but in our experience, if a baby isn't able to sleep well by the time teething starts, which is usually around five or six months of age, then she may be further from sleeping well than ever. This is because a human being of any age would have a difficult time undoing five months of bad habits, and here we're talking about a human being that is much harder to reason with.

Additionally, the child's parents, operating on five months of their own resultant sleep deprivation, are at this point running on fumes and making decisions as sound as those of a college freshman pulling an all-nighter before finals. They'll do anything to get some sleep, including things they previously vowed to never do, like bringing the child into bed with them. Or banning all sounds and lights in the house after a certain hour—mistakenly encouraging the fragile sleeping behavior rather than fixing it.

That's worst-case scenario stuff. If you haven't yet bought this book and are *still* standing in the bookstore considering the purchase, and that scenario scared you, good! Rest assured the good news is next.

We are happy to report that, in our experience, out of the thousands of parents who have followed the method laid out in the pages that follow, roughly 90 to 95 percent of their newborns were sleeping eight hours through the night by one month of age—and a majority of those achieved success within two weeks from the time training began. In the instances where success was elusive, it was almost always due to a significant underlying medical condition. (In Chapter 3, we also address some of the increasingly common GI issues that cause babies discomfort and distress, and create minor obstacles to our sleep training method, but which are usually overcome with your pediatrician's care.)

To be sure, we understand that there are parents out there who, for any number of reasons, may decide that they don't want their child sleeping through the night during the early weeks and months of life. Indeed, every aspect of parenting, from sleeping, feeding, and playing to educating, disciplining, and more, should be in accord with the parents' personal philosophies and values, goals and desires.

Parents should exercise their sovereign right to make their own decisions regarding the best interest of child and family. The Jassey Way is only one way to approach the sleep issue. Of course there are plenty of others, including the most commonly employed, laissez-faire approach, where the baby eventually "figures it out" on her own. We've heard of moms, and even some dads, who enjoy sitting up during the early morning hours, feeding baby or otherwise enjoying some alone time. It's probably obvious by now that we don't necessarily recommend that approach, but there's nothing inherently "wrong" with it.

The bottom line is that we want every family to be a happy and healthy family, and in our experience, the Jassey Way is a surer path to get there. But all families are different, and no approach could ever realistically be called *universal*. We would never begrudge parents their preference for raising a child.

You may also find that the Jassey Way may not be a good fit if you:

- Own a sizable stake in Starbucks or five-hour energy drinks.

- Have a bumper sticker that reads, "What Doesn't Kill Me Makes Me Stronger."

- Have ever said, "I'll get all the sleep I need when I'm dead," and not meant it as a joke.

The Jassey Way is unique in that it is designed for parents who wish to begin sleep training with their newborn shortly after birth—who want as few sleepless nights as is possible, and who don't want to give baby much of a chance to form bad sleeping habits.

Jassey Way babies are typically sleeping through the night weeks or months before most other sleep training methods even begin. Since we're veteran pediatricians, it should go without saying that we developed it within the framework of sound medical science—but, as you'll soon learn, we developed the core of it as an intuitive response to the unending cries for help from sleepless parents whose households and schedules had been upended before our very eyes.

If you want to nip that kind of trouble in the bud, read on. Then, pass this book to your spouse. Your joint success is more assured—and will come faster—if you're both reading from the same sheet of music.

And if your baby has already arrived and you're thinking, "I sure wish I'd read this before the baby was born," please *worry not*. The Jassey Way is also highly effective in getting infants to sleep, even if they're a bit older. Results may not come quite so rapidly, since an established routine (as chaotic as it may be) will need to be changed, but serenity can soon be yours as well.

THE "KINDNESS" OF STRANGERS

As you may have already experienced, parenting advice, both solicited and "volunteered," comes in abundance. New parents, wanting the perfect start for their little one, tend to listen intently and absorb all the information they can—perhaps too much of it. Whether it comes in the form of television programs, magazine articles, your own parents, their parents, family, friends, members of support groups, books, blogs, websites, infomercials, the inevitable playground note-comparing sessions with other parents, the cashier in the diner, the stranger in the elevator who insists on touching your belly, or whoever—and whatever—else, the whole world has an opinion ready-made for you. You know the expression "it takes a village to raise a child"? Most new parents will be lucky if the advice that's foisted on them comes from sources that number less than the population of a small country.

We have no doubt that nearly all of this advice is well intentioned. The challenge for the new parent is to determine which information is sound and helpful—medically and otherwise—and which is counterproductive.

There is a tremendous quantity of information out there, and parents—and pediatricians—must consider the *quality* of that information. Trusting the conventional wisdom can be unproductive, and sometimes even unhealthy or unsafe. Here's one well-known example: It wasn't too long ago that parents, even our own parents perhaps, used whiskey on the gums of teething babies. At some point, some intrepid person had to stand up and say, "Hey, maybe there are better, less hard liquor–based ways to deal with this crying issue. Just a thought, guys!"

We hope this book serves as a practical road map to a happy and healthy start for your family. One piece of conventional wisdom that sadly *is* true is that these years of bonding with and caring for baby will pass in the blink of an eye, leaving you with only warm memories.

It is our hope that by being well rested, you will create—and retain—even more of these warm memories.

CHAPTER ONE

Myths and Truths of Baby Sleep

First, a joke.

A guy goes to a dinner party. He introduces himself to the hostess, who's in the kitchen, cooking a roast. He notices that before she puts it in the oven, she cuts off the ends of the roast, puts it in the pan, and puts the pan in the oven.

"Out of curiosity," the man says, "why'd you cut off the ends of the roast?"

"That's the way my mother taught me," she says.

It turns out her mother is at the party, so the man follows up with her.

"Why do you cut off the ends of the roast?" he asks.

"That's the way my mother taught me," she says.

Turns out the grandmother's at the party, too. So the man goes up to her.

"That's the way my mother taught me," she says.

Amazingly, the very old great-grandmother is also at the party. So the man asks her.

"Why do you cut the ends off the roast?" he says.

"I had a very small roasting pan. I used to have to cut off the ends to make it fit in the pan."

When we talk about raising a baby nowadays, we're dealing with the same approach illustrated in that corny joke.

In this case, we're talking about the guiding beliefs of baby care, including "common wisdom" on issues like baby sleep and nutrition, that have been passed down from generation to generation, and along the way have assumed a mantle of *truth*.

In fact, just like the act of cutting off the ends of that roast, a lot of these guiding beliefs have no reason or logic behind them at all. As medical research progresses over time, best-parenting practices also evolve and are sometimes proven ineffective or even harmful.

We don't want you to start sleep training your little one while operating under any of these faulty assumptions or misinformation.

So let's take a look at a handful of common myths and outdated wisdom related to newborn diet and sleep—and let's clean them up . . .

MYTH: Newborns, practically by definition, turn households upside down and prevent the family from sleeping. The first months are exhausting and ridden with anxiety.

TRUTH: This is true for too many families, but it is by no means set in stone. The Jassey Way provides a practical and safe alternative, minimizing those dreaded sleepless nights and quickly allowing baby to enhance your life, not upend it. Informed parents can be confident in their ability to nurture the baby while simultaneously addressing the needs of the rest of the family.

MYTH: Most babies are just bad sleepers.

TRUTH: Most babies are able to sleep through the night, *if shown the way.* Habits—both good and bad—are formed early on. In most cases, when growing children are not able to achieve consistently sound sleep, it's because we, the parents, have inadvertently encouraged unhealthy sleep schedules. The Jassey Way is a simple, sound way of imparting to the baby healthy sleeping habits.

MYTH: Your mother and/or mother-in-law are pediatricians and baby experts.

TRUTH: Probably not.

MYTH: Rearing a child can be broken down into a science.

TRUTH: It's an art. No two experiences will be uniform, and adjustments will need to be made along the way.

MYTH: Most baby sleep books are meant to help parents train their children to develop healthy sleeping habits.

TRUTH: Most baby sleep books are actually meant to help parents train *themselves* to adopt a healthy attitude toward their baby's developing sleep habits. That might sound funny to you, but pick up most any baby sleep book and skim it and you'll see that this is true. They often address the *mom's* mental state, independent of what's going on with the child. That's why many of them recommend that Mom take steps that couldn't possibly influence her baby, like *telling* the infant that it's okay for her to go to sleep after she puts her in the crib every night. Or reassuring her that Mommy or Daddy will check in on her soon.

Most babies aren't born speaking fluent English, so who is Mom talking to in this scenario? Herself of course. We're all for a little talking to yourself if it helps you quiet your own emotions, but we won't pretend it's getting through to the baby.

This book will treat you, the parent, like the adult, and we'll leave all babying to, fittingly, your baby.

MYTH: If your baby is having trouble sleeping, you should wait until she's four months old and reaches a weight of fourteen pounds to start sleep training. That's when she'll be developmentally ready to self-soothe and sleep through the night.

TRUTH: This is another common misconception. First, there's no evidence that babies need to be a certain age or weight to begin sleep training. This isn't high school wrestling.

Secondly, the suggestion here is that parents should follow their baby's lead for a few months and expect that all of a sudden, at four months (or fourteen pounds), a magical switch will be flipped for the baby, and then she will start following *them*.

The truth is that the more a habit becomes ingrained in a

newborn, the harder it becomes to reverse that habit later on. They're no different than adults in this way.

Yes, it's certainly true that some infants will not have much trouble changing course at four months or later, as this myth suggests. But other infants will, and as we've said, it won't hurt *any* infant to try sleep training even earlier. By safely trying sleep training earlier, parents have nothing to lose and everything to gain.

MYTH: Nighttime feedings are necessary for infants.

TRUTH: They are not. What is necessary is that the baby gets enough to eat during a twenty-four-hour period. When and how frequently the nourishment is ingested is of no consequence as long as the baby gets the full day's supply.

MYTH: Letting a child cry at night leads to resentment and psychological damage.

TRUTH: This myth is rooted in visceral emotion and has absolutely no medical or scientific basis. Granted, no parent likes to hear his or her child cry. Even understanding that crying is a newborn's only mode of communication, it understandably can still be very tough to hear. But the reality is that crying in and of itself does no harm to baby. Understanding why exactly your baby may be crying—and having a levelheaded response to it—is far more productive than going to great lengths to avoid it altogether.

MYTH: When my baby cries, it's always because she is hungry.

TRUTH: Not true. Your baby may be hungry, but there are myriad other reasons she may be crying, such as teething, gastrointestinal discomfort, a dirty diaper, uncomfortable temperature, sickness, diaper rash or other pain, overtiredness (counterintuitive, but common), gas, the sound of a garbage truck outside, the phase of the moon, and so on.

You may have heard the saying "To a carpenter with a hammer, every problem looks like a nail." The most tangible tools parents have to soothe babies are the bottle and the breast, so it's no wonder every cry sounds like a hunger pang. This is simply not true and, as we'll discuss later on, may lead to bad habits.

MYTH: Babies cry to communicate to us that they don't like our attempts to change their routine. Crying is their way of protesting.

TRUTH: As we'll stress and reiterate time and again in this book, there are very few things that *all* babies do besides eating, crying, and pooping. A baby may cry because she doesn't like a particular change, she may cry because she's gassy, and she may cry just because. Most of the time, we will never know the reason. One thing we know is that, in reality, babies are more adaptable to change than most adults we know; virtually every waking second of their existence presents changes to their experience of the world. Sure, a particular baby may dislike a particular change, but babies don't "protest" change as a rule.

Do let us know if your baby takes up a picket sign and starts crawling around the perimeter of her crib while chanting slogans.

MYTH: Breast-fed babies must be fed eight to twelve times each day.

TRUTH: That's only true initially—until the breast milk comes in (engorgement), but after that, a more reasonable, less frequent schedule is not only possible, but more beneficial.

MYTH: Only the health of the baby matters during the first days and weeks of life. The rest of us are expendable, and it's heroic for parents to sacrifice their health and sanity in the service of coddling a newborn.

TRUTH: The baby's health during this early stage is important, of course. However, the health and welfare of the newborn's parents are *just as important*. Putting aside the emotional health of all involved for the moment, let's think about this rationally:

If a parent is run-down from sleep deprivation, he or she runs the risk of getting sick, which in turn can make the baby sick. Unfortunately, if a newborn develops a fever in the first six to eight weeks of life, it typically means automatic admission to the hospital, and potentially serious health risks.

We don't wish to scare you with any specifics, but rest assured that witnessing the battery of testing and invasive procedures that must be performed on a sick newborn is a harrowing experience the parent will not soon forget. To put the whole thing plainly, it's like the oxygen masks on planes; parents have to secure their own masks before they can properly take care of their child.

MYTH: When a baby gets older—say five or six months old—sleep training is often undone anyway, because at this stage the baby needs additional nourishment, making night feedings unavoidable.

TRUTH: This is another common misconception. If a child has been sleeping at night for months already, and is all of a sudden waking at night, it is unlikely to be due to hunger pangs. Children at this age are no more prone to these pangs than adults, since by this time their sleeping and eating cycles have been established. Night crying is still almost always due to an unrelated reason, most commonly teething. Making the mistake of reverting back to feeding at night has the very real potential of unraveling months of progress.

Incidentally, this book is not only about implementing the initial sleep training program; Chapter 6 also covers solutions for any number of events that might derail baby's previously sound sleeping habits. (These include teething, sickness, diaper rash, travel and proxy empathy if one parent is a fan of the New York Jets.)

CHAPTER TWO

The Jassey Way (Eat Right, Sleep Tight)

Parents' Bill of Rights

Article I: Sleep Training

1. Thoughtful sleep training, including our method, is perfectly safe for an infant at any age.

2. Sleep training is also healthy, because it helps keep parents well rested, alert and happy, and because it helps the baby develop the all-important skill of self-soothing—a skill that retains its infinite value over the course of an entire lifetime.

3. Accordingly, sleep training is by no means selfish on the part of parents. In fact, since its benefits to both baby and family are undeniable, we might say that not sleep training—and in the process allowing for a mutually needy dynamic between you and your baby—is a more selfish choice.

4. No two babies—even siblings—will respond to sleep training in exactly the same way. You must be careful not to sabotage yourself by judging your baby's progress on a curve based on another child.

5. Similarly, it's important not to let third party observers, including friends and family, derail you with unfounded critiques. And know that Internet message boards and comment sections are no substitution for established medical and scientific knowledge.

The Highly Abridged Jassey Way

The way to a man's heart is through his stomach.

—Proverb

If you only read one chapter in this book, it should be this one, because this is where we go over the Jassey Way in a *somewhat* step-by-step manner.

But, to simplify things even further, if you were to only read one *sentence* in this book, it should be this—let's call it the Golden Rule of the Jassey Way: *The longer a baby goes between feedings, the longer she'll be able to sleep.*

We'll get into the reasoning behind this in a moment, but in the way of evidence we offer the standard checklists that pediatricians use to track babies' development over the course of the first year of life. All of these checklists ask parents how frequently their baby feeds each day. Many if not most of them also ask how long the baby is sleeping per night. With most babies, you can see a straightforward correlation: *As time between feedings goes up, duration of sleep goes up.*

In fact, it was this very discovery that led us to develop the Jassey Way in the first place. It's a correlation that hides in plain sight, and yet so few parents and doctors seem to want to take advantage of it.

The Jassey Way Unabridged

We said we'd go over our method in a *somewhat* step-by-step manner, because, as you might have assumed by now, explaining any sleep training method in a straightforward chronological way is virtually impossible, because there are so many moving parts: baby, parents, milk, the different daily schedules of all involved, etc. As we've said before, taking care of a baby is more of an art than a science. To build on that analogy: Sleep training is more like building your own crib than putting together a crib from Ikea. Everyone will take the same general steps, and use the same general tools and supplies, but each family will have to tailor the steps to their particular needs. All this is to say that we don't want you to read this chapter as if you can only move on to step two after locking down step one, and can only move on to step three after locking down two. This is a *guide*; only you can know how to best implement it for your baby.

In our experience, the Jassey Way is not only a more effective way of getting your baby to sleep through the night; it's also an easier way. Still, we would never *promise* you that anything involving your baby will be easy; that's just unrealistic.

What we *can* promise you is that the Jassey Way is straightforward and, if not necessarily easy, *simple*. Because the whole operation is built on two simple baby principles:

1. For babies, feeding and sleeping are inseparable behaviors.

2. Babies are creatures of habit—so these two behaviors can be synchronized and harmonized. We can give them a *rhythm*.

The earlier we get your baby accustomed to a healthy eating and sleeping rhythm, the better for everyone involved.

WHY YOUR BABY WAKES UP

The primary reason your newborn will wake up during the night is hunger.* Put simply: When your baby is hungry, receptors in your baby's GI system tell your baby's brain, "We're hungry, you gotta feed us!" Naturally, if those receptors are triggered while your baby is asleep, your baby will wake up.

We are not saying that hunger is the *only* reason your baby might wake up during the night; just that it's the *most likely* reason.

The good news is that we can train those hunger receptors; we can get them used to a schedule, so that, as long as you're feeding your baby the daily amount necessary to enable healthy weight gain and development, they will not be triggered at arbitrary, inconvenient times.

....

* Additional reasons might include physical discomfort, loud noises, soft noises, plenty of other random occurrences.

To put it another way: If we can train your baby not to become hungry for an eight-hour stretch during the night, we will give your baby the best chance of *sleeping* through the night.

SYNCHRONIZING FEEDINGS

First things first: Conditioning your baby's digestive system, getting it into that rhythm we've been talking about, will not only help with sleep training; being a scheduled eater will improve your baby's temperament, provide your baby with a sense of security, and eliminate a lot of feeding guesswork—and the anxiety that comes with it—on your part. Everyone wins!

We want to train your baby to be an efficient feeder—allowing for a comfortable amount of time between feedings—and not to be a grazer.

Grazers have a much harder time when we try to get them to sleep through the night.

Note: We've heard moms say that their babies should feed more frequently than the rate we recommend simply because when they are fed more frequently, they finish every last drop. That might be true, but it doesn't mean it's necessarily healthy for the baby. A baby's innate reflex is to suck; sucking doesn't always mean the baby is hungry.

To be sure, one of the first reflexes a baby is able to exercise in utero is sucking. When Mom gets a level 2 ultrasound at around twenty-one to twenty-two weeks into her pregnancy, one of the very first things the sonographer will point out to her on-screen is the action of the baby sucking. It's a primitive reflex that babies use to, among other things, soothe themselves.

All this is to say that babies like to exercise their sucking muscles a lot, and sure, they'll do so when milk is given to them. But that doesn't mean they need to eat to self-soothe. In fact, they shouldn't eat to self-soothe at all.

Now let's state the obvious: Your baby needs a certain amount of milk per day, or twenty-four-hour period, to maintain healthy weight gain and development. We'll talk about determining that number later on, but for now, suffice it to say that it's usually somewhere around 2.25 ounces per pound of body weight. Every day, it's your job as a parent to feed your baby roughly that amount (excepting the inevitable spit-ups, temporary refusals, and other little setbacks). It doesn't matter if it's two ounces every two hours, or four ounces every four hours, as long as the total is the same at the end of the day. Contrary to too-popular belief: When and how frequently you feed your baby that amount is almost entirely up to you—not your baby.

That's an important point, worth repeating: It's your job as a parent to feed your baby in a healthy manner. It sounds strange to say, but one of your duties is not to let your baby distract you from doing that job.

There are two main reasons that you should dictate feedings to your baby, and not the other way around:

1. Sometimes your baby will cry, or send another signal that could be interpreted as hunger, at a time when she is hungry and when it would indeed be healthy to feed her. But other times, your baby will send you such "signals" when feeding is not at all necessary. She's a baby! Her signals

can often get scrambled, and your ability to interpret them can, too.

In short, letting your baby dictate feedings is a case of the blind leading the blind.

2. If you let your baby dictate the feeding schedule by crying, or whatever other signals you can't help but respond to, you give up too much control over a behavior that can become unmanageable in a hurry. Before you know it, you'll be feeding at erratic times, feeling as if you're feeding all day long without any breaks, potentially running out of milk if you're breast-feeding, and generally worrying yourself sick over calorie intake, keeping up with the demand, and more. And you might well be miserably tired while all this is going on. Then, before you know it, your newborn is six months old and the bad habits are so ingrained that climbing out of them will seem like scaling the Grand Canyon— while you're sleep-deprived.

THE BOTTOM LINE

It's not just that you *can* regulate your baby's feedings. It's that you *should* regulate your baby's feedings.

Our goal is to structure your baby's feedings so that they come in consistent amounts, at consistent intervals—to synchronize them to a schedule that's best for your baby and your family.

Generally speaking, we want to get your baby feeding every four hours over the course of the day, with the final feeding keeping your baby satisfied for seven or eight hours overnight—a total of five feedings over a twenty-four-hour period.

For example: One commonly employed schedule comprises feeding the baby at 7 a.m., 11 a.m., 3 p.m., 7 p.m., and 11 p.m., after which the baby will sleep for around seven or eight hours, bringing you back to the 7 a.m. feeding. (Before too long, as your baby's digestive system continues to mature, the final feeding can be eliminated, and the number of hours your baby is able to sleep through the night without interruption may even reach double digits.)

As we've said, babies are creatures of habit. So once your baby is accustomed to a schedule like this, she will remain accustomed to it. She will rely on it.

SYNCHRONIZING THE DAY—DAY BY DAY

We can't get the night right without first getting the day right.

We have found that the ideal time between *daytime* feedings—in terms of enabling both healthy weight gain and development *and* peaceful sleep—is generally around four hours.

If you and your baby are already on such a schedule, then you can probably skip ahead to the next section, Owning the Night.

If not . . . keep reading.

If Your Baby Is Used to Going Longer
Than Four Hours Between Feedings

If your baby is accustomed to waiting *longer* between feedings—say, five hours—we recommend cutting those intervals down so they're closer to four hours. A daily schedule that contains some five-hour periods between feedings is probably perfectly healthy for weight gain and development if the baby seems comfortable with it. But in our experience, those babies don't end up sleeping for an extended stretch at night as easily as the "four-hour babies." This might be because human beings are only equipped to go without food for one extended stretch per day. Whatever the case, we find that four hours between feedings works best for sleep training.

If Your Baby Is Used to Going Fewer Than Four Hours Between Feedings

If your baby is accustomed to feeding *under* every four hours during the day, we recommend widening the time between feedings by fifteen minutes per feeding, per day (twenty-four-hour period).

For instance, if you've been feeding every three hours, on the first day of "stretching out," you'll feed every three hours and fifteen minutes. If you've been feeding every two and a half hours, on the first day you'll widen that to two hours and forty-five minutes.

We promise you that that extra fifteen minutes is not going to harm your baby. Your baby may cry, but she won't pop a blood vessel or develop a hernia or a facial tic.

Nor will she grow up to resent you when she's older. (Except when she's a teenager; no one has solved that yet.)

And while we need you to stick it out through those fifteen-minute intervals and not *feed* your baby, we absolutely recommend soothing your baby in other ways. Pick her up, hold her, sing to her, do what you need to do. Just don't feed her.

You can do it! We believe in you.

On Day Two, you'll expand the time between feedings by

another fifteen minutes. So if you were at three hours between feedings originally, and went to 3:15 the first day, you should be at 3:30 on the second day.

And on and on, adding fifteen minutes per feeding per day, day after day, until you've reached four hours between feedings. At this point, you'll be feeding your baby around four times during the daytime.

Two things to note:

- We recommend increasing the time between feedings by fifteen minutes per day simply because we've found that it's an interval that's generally easy for baby and Mom to handle.

- But by no means do you have to *limit* the increases to fifteen minutes per feeding per day. You could try twenty or thirty minutes if you like.

You can always go slower, too. You can make it a goal to increase these intervals by fifteen minutes every two or three days, rather than every day, if you feel more comfortable that way. Or you can increase them by five or ten minutes per day, if you'd like. It will probably take a bit longer to reach the ultimate goal in those cases, but some progress is much more preferable than none—and still should do the trick in the long run.

As always, use your best judgment. Ultimately, you're the only one who can know what's best for your baby, and you're the one assessing the results in real time.

If your baby happens to be sleeping when the four-hour mark hits, you should gently wake her up to make sure she feeds. Remember, we're trying to get on a schedule here—there's no "reward" for going more than four hours between feedings during the daytime. It only risks interfering with the rest of the schedule. Additionally, we don't want your baby to get her days and nights confused, or to risk turning her into a nocturnal creature, by letting her sleep for an extended stretch during the day.

Here is a sample feeding schedule in which the time between feedings, originally set at three hours, is increased by fifteen minutes per day:

DAY "ZERO":	8 a.m. →	11 a.m. →	2 p.m. →	5 p.m. →	8 p.m. →	11 p.m.
DAY ONE:	8 a.m. →	11:15 a.m. →	2:30 p.m. →	5:45 p.m. →	9 p.m. →	12:15 a.m.
DAY TWO:	8 a.m. →	11:30 a.m. →	3 p.m. →	6:30 p.m. →	10 p.m.*	
DAY THREE:	8 a.m. →	11:45 a.m. →	3:30 p.m. →	7:15 p.m. →	11 p.m.	
DAY FOUR:	8 a.m. →	12 p.m. →	4 p.m. →	8 p.m. →	**12 a.m.**	

Note: At first glance, it may look like only the 11 a.m. feeding is extended by fifteen minutes each day, and that the others are extended more. But that's not the case.

Rather, each fifteen-minute delay builds on the ones before it, to push back the scheduled *time* of each successive feeding. But not the time *between feedings*.

In other words, the time of the third feeding on Day One has to take into account the fact that the second feeding came fif-

---

* Ideally, if you're lucky, you won't need to feed after the 10 p.m. feeding on Day Two until a reasonable hour the next morning. But this can be a slightly tricky period, where you'll have to play it by ear a little. In the next section, we give you a strategy for dealing with this transition phase.

teen minutes later than the day before. So even though the baby fed at 2 p.m. on Day Zero and 2:30 p.m. the next day, she did not wait an extra thirty minutes for that feeding; 11:15 a.m. (second feeding) to 2:30 p.m. (third feeding) is only three hours and fifteen minutes, not three and a half hours.

The fifteen-minute additions accumulate over the course of the day until the final feeding comes a full hour later than it did the *day* before. But it's still only three hours and fifteen minutes from the *feeding* before.

Owning the Night

THE TRANSITION PHASE

Stretching out the nighttime is, of course, a little different. Now we're aiming to have a single interval between feedings—the final feeding of the night and the first morning feeding the next day—lasting seven or eight hours.

But the thing is, until your baby is sleeping seven to eight hours through the night, you're effectively in a transitional phase. And during this phase, the timing of your feedings—especially that one right before bed—might be a little off every single night.

Most people like that final feeding to be between 10 and 12 p.m., so the baby can sleep until around 6 to 8 a.m., and allow *them* to have a normal night's sleep.

Some parents might naturally fall into a pattern where they start the day by feeding anywhere between 7 and 8 a.m., and if they're near our four-hour ideal, the rest of the day unfolds smoothly:

7 a.m. → 11 a.m. → 3 p.m. → 7 p.m. → 11 p.m.... → 6–7 a.m. next morning

or

8 a.m. → 12 p.m. → 4 p.m. → 8 p.m. → midnight ... → 7–8 a.m. next morning

Parents who settle into feeding schedules similar to the ones above might be able to achieve that seven- or eight-hour overnight stretch a little more easily. As when a plane is landing on a runway directly in front of it, everything's already lined up; they won't have to move that final feeding back or forth much.

THE TRICKY TIME

But other parents won't be quite so lucky. After increasing the time between daytime feedings to every four hours, their "natural" schedule might end up placing that sleep runway closer to 1 a.m.:

DAY "ZERO":	9 a.m. →	12 p.m. →	3 p.m. →	6 p.m. →	9 p.m. →	12 a.m.
DAY ONE:	9 a.m. →	12:15 p.m. →	3:30 p.m. →	6:45 p.m. →	10 p.m.	
DAY TWO:	9 a.m. →	12:30 p.m. →	4 p.m. →	7:30 p.m. →	11 p.m.	
DAY THREE:	9 a.m. →	12:45 p.m. →	4:30 p.m. →	8:15 p.m. →	12 a.m.	
DAY FOUR:	9 a.m. →	1 p.m. →	5 p.m. →	9 p.m. →	**1 a.m.**	

Most parents are not going to want to settle into a schedule where the final feeding comes around 1 a.m.; it's simply too late for them to get the sleep *they* need.

But for their part, most infants are not going to be able to go from 9 p.m. to your ideal wake-up time the next morning, even if it's pretty early, like 6 a.m. That's too long a stretch to ask of newborns. So we can't *cut out* a feeding. They'll need to feed one more time during the night—specifically, at a very inconvenient time, somewhere between 1 and 3 a.m. Not only do you want to not have to wake up around then, but that would mess up the next day's schedule, leading to a vicious cycle.

At the same time, it's difficult to squeeze in an earlier feeding—around midnight or earlier—because if your baby fed around 9 p.m., she might not *be able* to take milk before midnight.

You're stuck between a rock and a hard place. What do you do?

As a general rule, we recommend trying to get the seven to eight hours of uninterrupted night sleep established and settled *before* homing in on that ideal final feeding time.

This means aiming for a second-to-last (penultimate) feeding no later than 8 p.m., so you can have a final feeding no later than midnight, and at least have a realistic shot at not having to feed until around 6 the next morning.

Here's where it gets even trickier. Please bear with us for a moment:

In order to arrive at an 8 p.m. feeding, you might have to *reduce* the time between the other feedings. We know we've spent the rest of this chapter begging you to go in the other direction—stretching feedings *out*—but for the sake of giving your baby the best shot at that seven- to eight-hour stretch of night sleep, we're okay with a little "cheating" for a few days.

Here's what we mean.

If you fed at or around 9 a.m., and if you're going four hours between feedings, by simple math you're going to arrive at a 9 p.m. feeding (or maybe even later).

In order to rein in that 9 p.m. feeding, in order to bring it back to 8 p.m. or earlier, you start the first feeding of the day fifteen minutes earlier, and aim for 3:45 between feedings after that, instead of the usual four hours.

Over the course of four feedings, this small adjustment should amount to shifting that 9 p.m. feeding back by close to an hour:

Instead of feedings going like this:

9 a.m. → 1 p.m. → 5 p.m. → 9 p.m.

They'll go like this:

8:45 a.m. → 12:30 p.m. → 4:15 p.m. → **8 p.m.**

(Now the very last, before-bed feeding can come at midnight or earlier.)

Obviously, these times are just estimates, rough guidelines. To some extent, you're on your own when figuring out these adjustments; every family's situation is unique.

But beyond your specific situation, you can see how a minor modification during the day can help you avoid that booby trap that lies between 10 and 12 p.m.—the trap that inevitably leads to our archenemy, the middle-of-the-night feeding.

This also makes clear why we recommend prioritizing the stretch of night sleep over the four-hour daytime intervals, and the ideal final feeding time: Making some minor tweaks in your baby's daytime behavior will always be easier than "fixing" the middle-of-the-night feeding if she gets used to it. So we want to steer clear of that 1 to 3 a.m. feeding essentially at all costs, including our four-hour ideal.

It goes without saying that, during this transitional phase, negotiating that final feeding is going to take some ad-libbing and adjusting on the fly on your part.

The transition might take a few days; it may take a few weeks. During this time, your feedings might be "off" a bit every night.

Again, use your best judgment. We can give you the general lay of the land, a broad map that points out key destinations. But it's up to you to find the particular routes that are right for you.

Whatever you do, whatever day-to-day successes and setbacks you experience while sleep training your baby, remember: It's all perfectly okay, as long as you're generally sticking to our first rule of going in the right direction, *stretching out* the time between feedings.

STICK THE LANDING (THE FINAL FEEDING)

It's important to wake the baby for the final feeding if she is sleeping—even if you think she might sleep "through the night." Yes, at that point in the evening, she may well sleep a total of seven hours—but if it's the seven hours from 8 p.m. to 3 a.m., and you have to wake up at that awful hour, what good does it do you?

Again, it's all about synchronizing the feedings to a schedule that is healthy for both your baby *and* your family.

You may even want to add half an ounce to that final feeding before bed. We call this the "turkey feeding," since it's inspired by the lethargy we feel after gorging ourselves on Thanksgiving.

DREAM FEEDING

If, despite your best attempts, your baby doesn't wake up for that final feeding, try to "dream feed" her. Babies are born with a powerful sucking instinct (as noted earlier), and you can take advantage of that; most babies will feed even while dozing.

In order to safely dream feed your baby, hold her upright while she feeds, so that if the milk goes down the wrong pipe, she's in no danger of asphyxiating.

SOME MINOR ADJUSTMENTS

Since widening the time between feedings will necessarily increase the amount of milk your baby needs *per feeding* (so that you can maintain the necessary daily total), you'll need to adjust accordingly. This is simpler than it might sound.

Try to figure out how many feedings you'll be eliminating in a given day (it won't be more than one or two), and then divide that amount of food over the remaining feedings. By way of explanation, let's say you give your baby two ounces of milk per feeding, and due to the widening between feedings, you're reducing the total number of that day's feedings by one. Now you effectively have two ounces "left over" or, to put it another way, two ounces you have to "make up" to reach that day's total.

If the day's schedule called for four total feedings, you'd divide two ounces by four to find the added amount *per feeding*: 0.5 ounce.

Bedtime Routine

Some of the other major sleep training methods emphasize the need to have a consistent "bedtime routine." As we say time and again in this book, we place a great deal of value on *consistency*. So we agree; it's good to have a little bedtime routine for both you and your baby to rely on. But for our part, we'd like to emphasize the *little* part. We don't think it's necessary to design a lengthy program that proceeds from room to room with the type of choreography that's usually reserved for a royal wedding processional and ends with placing your baby in her crib like you're trying to set an egg down on a basketball.

In the end, the purpose of establishing a bedtime routine, in addition to adding to the consistency of your baby's young life, is to establish the difference between night and day. As long as you bear that guideline in mind when getting your child ready for bed, you'll be providing enough routine.

Around an hour before bedtime, begin to wind things down. Dim or turn off any bright lights, eliminate any loud noises, and scale all physical activity with your baby down to the "gentle" and "light" levels. You don't have to do these things at *precisely* the same time, or in the same order, every night, any more than you need to brush your teeth and wash your face at the same time every night. So long as you wind things down, you'll be fine; they don't have to be wound down in precisely the same order.

Once your baby is in the bassinet or crib, you can read to her, or sing to her, or read song lyrics to her, or softly sing your favorite book passages to her—whatever you find enjoyable and effective.

If you want to go the highly choreographed route for your bedtime routine, that's perfectly fine, too. We're not advising *against* that, and some parents might prefer to rely on that themselves. It's certainly not harmful.

We like to stress that such routines are not strictly *necessary* only because we don't want you to overthink or stress out about it unnecessarily.

Just remember to set the right mood around an hour before bedtime.

OWNING THE NIGHT

For many of you, this is where the rubber meets the road—overnight, when we want you and your baby to be sleeping at the same time.

Undoubtedly, in the beginning, your baby will wake up at some point during the night and cry—and you will want to feed her.

But you shouldn't. Not if you want to harmonize your baby's sleeping and eating, so that your baby's on a schedule that's healthy for her, and the rest of your family.

By now, you've almost certainly learned about the "cry it out" method, the "no cry" method, the "least cry" method and various other strategies for soothing your baby if she cries during the night.

We advocate a very straightforward approach: If your baby wakes up crying during the night, try to soothe her as best you know how—without *instinctually* looking to feeding her.

Pick her up, rock her, sing to her, coo to her; do what feels natural.

But try not to feed her—*at least until you've made it fifteen minutes longer since the last feeding than you did the previous night.*

If you've already fed your baby the total amount of milk necessary per day to enable healthy weight gain and development, your baby will be just fine without an overnight feeding. Period. End of story.

We Understand!

WE UNDERSTAND that your baby might, effectively, raise holy hell.

WE UNDERSTAND that this can be painful to hear. We've been there; we have five daughters between us.

WE UNDERSTAND the feeling that holding your baby, or rocking your baby, or any other non-feeding attempt at soothing might feel insufficient.

WE UNDERSTAND the urge to feed in these situations can be strong, and even overwhelming.

In your moments of extreme doubt, please read the boldfaced statement below. Repeat it to yourself like a mantra. Cling to it like a life preserver in a stormy sea. (You will find more advice on crying in Chapter 3.)

Know that you're playing the long game on behalf of your baby, not grasping for your own quick fix. Never forget: *This overnight crying is more difficult for you than for your baby.* Don't sacrifice what are actually your baby's best interests to, in reality, soothe yourself.

Don't Play Ping-Pong

If it's the middle of the night, and all your soothing attempts (or tricks) don't seem to pacify your baby's crying—if you've done all you could humanly do and it just hasn't worked—and you absolutely *have* to get to bed yourself, try to stick it out for at least fifteen minutes, and *then* feed your baby. Then, the following night, make it your goal to stick it out fifteen minutes or, if possible, a half hour longer.

For instance, if your baby slept from midnight to 3 a.m. before waking up, and waking you up, try to hold her, rock her, sing to her, or calm her another way until at least 3:15 before feeding. Then, the next night, make sure you stretch it out until at least 3:45 or even 4 a.m. Ideally, you won't feed overnight at all, but if you must, making *some* progress is better than making none.

It's crucial to go in one direction—making these intervals *longer*—even if incrementally, as opposed to "ping-ponging" (one night going longer, the next going shorter, etc.). As creatures of habit, babies run the risk of becoming accustomed to an erratic schedule in the same way that they can come to rely on a consistent one.

Breast-Feeding

As we said earlier, we do not endorse formula feeding over breast-feeding, or breast-feeding over formula feeding; we endorse whatever Mom and Dad feel most comfortable with.

Just bear in mind that it will take a bit more time to adopt the Jassey Way when breast-feeding than it will with formula feeding—for two basic reasons:

- Many studies and experts have suggested that babies digest breast milk more quickly than formula.* So your baby might not be able to go as long between feedings of breast milk as she would between feedings of the same amount of formula. In other words, there might be less "wiggle room" when trying to stretch out breast feedings.

- It generally takes eight to twelve feedings to kick-start the milk engine and get breast milk going consistently, so you'll have to get over that hump before beginning sleep training.

Still, once you are able to rely on the milk supply from your breast, or once you are able to pump consistently, the Jassey Way should play out the same as it does with formula feeding.

THE JASSEY WAY AND BREAST MILK

The Jassey Way, at heart, works the same whether Mom is breast- or formula-feeding. There are only two minor differences be-

---

* Babies may digest breast milk more quickly, but in our eyes, this has not been definitively proven—especially in light of the fact that formulas continue to evolve, and more closely resemble the molecular structure of breast milk all the time. Nowadays the major commercial formulas contain EPA and DHA (key fatty acids found in breast milk); they have the same amount of calories as breast milk; and they have relatively the same amount of sodium chloride.

tween the two approaches in the context of our method of sleep training: the initial "ramp up" stage, and the manner in which the amount of milk per feeding is measured.

Ramping Up

As we said, Mom needs to get baby on the breast eight to twelve times to get consistent milk in. But once the milk is consistent, you're ready to start the Jassey Way.

If you are planning to pump breast milk and feed via bottle, once that consistent milk is in, you can begin the Jassey Way just as if you were formula feeding.

If you are going to breast-feed your baby directly, keep the following in mind.

Measuring Quantity: Time Takes Precedent over Ounces

As we stressed earlier, the Jassey Way is heavily dependent on your baby receiving precisely the goal amount of milk per day—with no more or less, if you can help it.

If you're formula feeding from a bottle, or feeding breast milk from a bottle, reaching that goal amount is a pretty straightforward proposition. But breast-feeding directly makes it slightly more nuanced.

Of course, you can pump milk when the breast is full to gauge how much milk is in each feeding, but that amount is bound to fluctuate over time, so we'd just as soon measure according to time rather than volume.

That is to say, an efficient breast-feeding baby—one that feeds every four hours during the day—should feed approximately fifteen to twenty minutes on each side, per feeding.

Those that feed every two hours during the day will take around five to ten minutes on each side.

Both of these feeding rates—every two hours and every four hours—should reach the goal number of calories. But as we've established, feeding more often usually leads to choppier sleep at night.

Note: Once your baby is sleeping through the night, Mom's milk production will usually follow the infant's schedule. But for a brief period, some moms might have to wake up and pump milk at night before their body clock adjusts. This transition is usually temporary and won't be necessary for more than a few nights.

For more information on breast-feeding, please read Chapter 5, "Of Breast and Bottle."

Common Mistakes

Everyone has a plan—until they get punched in the mouth.

—Former heavyweight boxing champion Mike Tyson, evaluating strategies his opponents might use to beat him in the ring

We probably wouldn't hold up Mike Tyson as a parenting expert, but we like that quote for describing how difficult a crying baby can be for parents. You can read every great baby book there is, get the measured advice of every wise person you know, map out a studied, detailed plan for dealing with any issue that might arise with your baby, and then the infant starts crying and all your preparation goes out the window. In other words, in Tyson parlance, crying can be a punch in the face. In fact, the analogy might not be as symbolic as it seems; we've heard many moms describe the sound of their baby crying as painful or even excruciating.

In the next chapter, "The Crying Game," we'll discuss in detail why baby crying is, in most cases, nothing to get upset about. But for our purposes right now, we briefly want to call your attention to crying because, in our experience, it tends to be the main culprit when our sleep training method doesn't succeed.

Just as the Jassey Way is relatively simple and straightforward, so too can it be derailed by a couple of relatively simple missteps—both of which revolve around the baby's crying.

Here are the two most common impediments to the correct implementation and overall success of our sleep method, in our experience.

THE BRIBE

My mother comes over all the time, and when the baby's crying, she'll say, "Just feed her." But I'm the one who's going to be kept up at night, not her.

—Jessica S., mom

"The Bribe" is a term we've coined to refer to the action of giving a baby the breast or bottle to quell a crying spell when you're between scheduled feedings.

We've seen many parents who don't realize how much they feed their babies, essentially inadvertently, just by reaching for the bottle or the breast reflexively, almost out of habit. As we said before (and will say again), *as long as your baby is getting enough calories per feeding—and per day—she's likely not crying out of hunger or pain, and any subsequent feeding only serves to disrupt sleep training.* But even when parents understand this, the instinct to feed their baby is so automatic that it doesn't register as violating the sleep plan.

At the same time, if your baby cries in the middle of the night and shows no signs of stopping, you might consciously want to administer the Bribe feeding, so you can go back to sleep yourself. Maybe you have an important day tomorrow, and you simply can't afford to wait your baby out on this particular night. Or maybe, for whatever reason, you just can't take it anymore, and you feel that if your infant doesn't stop crying, you'll go permanently insane—for *real*—and so you give her the milk.

We don't blame anyone for any of this. Life happens, so to speak. We don't expect anyone to blindly sacrifice the other important parts of their life for the sake of sleep training. That wouldn't help anyone in the long run.

Remember: You don't need to operate as if you're running the kitchen in a hotel with twenty-four-hour, round-the-clock room service, and your baby is a cranky guest who keeps the phone ringing off the hook. The kitchen *can* close.

Your job is to be more like the proprietor of a good clean bed-and-breakfast. You provide delicious and nutritious meals, but they don't come *on demand.*

A FINAL WARNING ABOUT THE MIDDLE-OF-THE-NIGHT BOTTLE:

THE LOSS OF FAITH

If the most common impediment to the Jassey Way is a mom or dad losing nerve *in the moment* and feeding a crying baby off-schedule, the second most common misstep is a parent losing his or her faith in the method as a whole and giving up on the whole thing before it's had a real chance to work.

As we've said, babies are all different, and every baby will respond to sleep training—our method *or any other*—differently.

You could be one of the lucky ones who sees their baby take to sleep training like a young Beyoncé took to dance lessons, and sleeping through the night in just a few days. As you can read in Chapter 9, that scenario does happen; we see it all the time. That's not to say it's necessarily *common*—just that it's not *un*common.

(In fact, in our experience, when parents diligently apply the Jassey Way, in most cases the child *does* start sleeping at least seven hours overnight within a week or so.)

But maybe your work with sleep training will require a bit more patience, with the child gradually giving you more and more time of uninterrupted sleep each night, and reaching seven or eight hours in around two or three weeks, or even a month. The key in that scenario is to accept that the progress is going to be gradual and not to give up—not to lose faith in the method just because it didn't bring *immediate* success.

It's also important to keep in mind that sometimes a baby will take two steps forward and one step back; you have to trust in the method after the occasional backslide. Measure success over several days at a time, not according to a single day by itself.

The Small Sacrifice vs. the Large Sacrifice

Baby sleep training, like anything else in life that holds the potential for a spectacular payoff, requires some degree of sacrifice. The Jassey Way requires you to abstain from auto-feeding your baby when she cries, and it may require you to "wait her out" over the course of a few sleepless nights.

The good news is that those sacrifices all come up-front. Once your baby *is* getting consistently good overnight sleep, there isn't any sacrifice necessary to maintain it.

But if you *did* give up on sleep training too soon—if you *did* lose faith—think of the long-term sacrifice you'd be making for the sake of that quick, in-the-moment fix. You'd be sacrificing not just nights, not just weeks, but *months* of good, consistent, restful and restorative sleep—for the whole family, along with the chance for your child to learn the essential skill of self-soothing sooner rather than later.

In this way, we can frame the question of whether or not to sleep train as a question of sacrifices: Would you rather sacrifice a little up-front, or sacrifice a great deal in the long run?

For a wider perspective on the sacrifices, challenges and, most important, benefits and rewards of sleep training, please go to Chapter 4, "What's the Big Deal About All This Anyway?" and Chapter 9, "Parent Testimonials," which presents first-person accounts of sleep training from real parents on the front lines.

That's It

That's it. That's the Jassey Way. That's the written, all-inclusive, unabridged version of the spiel we've given to thousands of new moms and dads over the past couple of decades—and the one we'll continue to give for decades to come.

And it's the system we used with all five of our own daughters and that, God willing, they'll use with their children.

We're that confident in it.

We realize that implementing our method might at times be

difficult for you. We wouldn't recommend it if it wasn't more than worth it.

MATH!

Our goal in this book is to help your baby sleep through the night, for the benefit of the whole family. This book is not about how *much* your baby should be consuming per day to enable healthy weight gain and development; you'll no doubt have determined that number previously.

Nevertheless, we'd be negligent if we didn't include the way we calculate that daily amount.

Our formula:

Baby weight in pounds × 2.25 = Total number of ounces per day

So, let's say your baby weighs eight pounds:

8 × 2.25 = 18 ounces of milk per day

In order to apply the ideal Jassey Way feeding schedule of five feedings per day to the goal of eighteen ounces of milk per day, we divide eighteen ounces by five:

18 ÷ 5 = 3.6 OUNCES PER FEEDING

Please understand that the math we just presented is a rough framework intended to help you find your baby's sleeping and eating "sweet spots."

But every child is different, and every child's metabolism is different. What works for one baby weighing 6 pounds, 14 ounces may not be as ideal for another baby weighing 6 pounds, 14 ounces.

Only you and your pediatrician can know what's best for your particular little one. As always, use your best judgment, in consultation with your doctor.

Don't Let the Numbers Drive You Nuts

During his residency, Lewis used to tell parents, "You have to do thirteen ounces a day" (or fourteen, or fifteen, etc.). But one time one set of parents came to him and told him that at the end of the day, their child had been half an ounce short of the target amount of milk, and in trying to force-feed her that final half ounce, they had caused her to throw up all the milk from her previous bottle—so she ended up even *further* from the target amount.

We know that these milk ratio formulas can "drive parents crazy," and if some of them would rather "feel it out" on a daily basis, that's absolutely fine.

As long as a baby is consistently filling her diapers with both liquid and solid waste, and as long as the baby's mouth is consistently moist, you can be sure that baby is getting the proper amount of nutrients on a daily basis—perhaps even more than the proper amount. Just make sure to look out for those signs.

Whatever you do, don't get *hung up* on these formulas. If you end up being off by a few ounces, in either direction, everything will still be fine.

So either route—strictly sticking to the numbers, or ballparking it while monitoring your baby's progress—will get you where you want to go, namely meeting your baby's nutritional needs.

Remember, you're not alone in this process. For one thing, you will be bringing your baby in for monthly checkups, during which your doctor will weigh your baby and plot that weight on a growth chart. If your baby's growth is following the proper curve of height and weight, you'll know your feedings are on the money. If your baby is off the curve, your doctor will help you make the adjustments to get her back on it.

While it can feel stressful and complex, in reality, figuring out how much to feed the baby is something that *billions* of parents have gone through before you.

And we're all still here. That should tell you something.

Going the Distance (Getting 10+ Hours)

Once your baby has been getting seven or eight hours of uninterrupted sleep per night for at least a few weeks in a row, you might want to get a little greedy by extending it to eleven or even twelve hours. This is not necessary per se, but a lot of parents will take it if they can get it.

Some babies might naturally start to sleep longer after four months of age, but that's not something that should be taken for granted. Additionally, around six to ten months of age (but as early as three), babies start teething, which often leads to a regression in sleep behavior; it's nice to have some extra "insurance" hours in the baby bank.

At this point, you won't be surprised to learn that we're going to stretch seven or eight hours of overnight sleep into eleven or twelve hours by small, daily increments. The main difference is that whereas we were previously trying to gain fifteen minutes per feeding per day, now we're going to go for thirty total minutes— fifteen on the front end, and fifteen on the back end.

In other words, if your baby typically wakes up at 6 a.m. and you feed her, now try not feeding her until at least 6:15. That's what we mean by extending the "back end"—it's simply the first feeding after your baby wakes up.

Obviously the "front end" refers to the last feeding of the night, before your baby goes to sleep. Let's say your baby takes the last feeding and is in bed by 10 p.m. Try pushing that back to 9:45 p.m.

The next day, try adding another fifteen minutes on both ends. Finish the last feeding by 9:30 p.m., and delay the first feeding the next morning to 6:30 a.m.

Please keep in mind that this thirty-minute-per-day increase is just a suggestion. We've found that this is a good increment for most of the families we've worked with. But you might prefer to go ten minutes in both directions at a time, or five, or twenty. As always, it's what you feel comfortable with. It's about using your best judgment and seeing what works for your child.

It's also important to note that, for whatever reason, you may prefer or find it easier to add time to *only* the front or back end each night. That's fine, too. We recommend adding to both ends because in our experience babies go along with it with relative ease, but again, there is never any one-size-fits-all rule.

Eventually, if you keep adding time to the front end, you're not just going to add time to your baby's overnight sleep; you're also going to eliminate a feeding. It's unavoidable.

For instance, let's say you start out with the "ideal" feeding schedule we use as an example so much in this book:

8 a.m. → 12 p.m. → 4 p.m. → 8 p.m. → 12 a.m.

Then, let's say that after a week or so, you cut an hour and a half off of that front end:

8 a.m. → 12 p.m. → 4 p.m. → 8 p.m. → **10:30 p.m.**

If your baby fed at 8 p.m., and now you've worked your way back, and you've extended that front end so that she's going to sleep around 10:30 p.m., there's a good chance she's not going to be at all hungry before bedtime.

For a long time, she relied on four hours between daytime feedings; that's the Jassey Way in action. Then you cut into the front end—her last feeding before bed—so that it scaled back from around midnight to around 11:45 p.m., to around 11:30, and so on. At many of those intervals, feeding before bed might have come easily to your baby, even if it was less than four hours since the last feeding. The difference between four hours and three hours and forty-five minutes and three and a half hours might have been negligible to her. You can play around with that final feeding in order to see what works best.

But at some point, maybe three hours or less—who can predict?—she might cross a threshold where eating so soon after the last feeding is just not possible.

At that point, we recommend eliminating that last feeding altogether. So now, the daily schedule would look like this:

8 a.m. → 12 p.m. → 4 p.m. → 8 p.m. → ~~10:30 p.m.~~

If 8 p.m. (or whenever that feeding comes on your schedule) is not your ideal time for the final feeding, for whatever reason, you can always temporarily adjust the other feedings in the day to land on the time that *is* best for you and the infant. By now, your baby should be a good enough sleeper that temporarily adjusting the times between those earlier feedings—for the sake of nailing down the time of your ideal final feeding—should not be a problem.

For example, if you were on the 8 a.m., 12 p.m., 4 p.m., 8 p.m. schedule, but you'd like the last feeding to be at 9 p.m., you can adjust accordingly by temporarily breaking the four-hour rule. You can feed at 8 a.m., 12:30 p.m., 5 p.m., and 9 p.m. for a few days, to get her used to taking that last feeding at 9. Then after a few days you can "realign" those earlier feedings.

It's all very variable, obviously. A little ad-libbing is inevitable in any successful sleep training.

Now your baby is feeding four times a day, instead of five, so you'll have to add a little bit of milk to each feeding to reach the total daily nutritional goal.

In order to figure out how much milk to add to each feeding, divide the number of ounces of the missing feeding by four, the new number of feedings.

For instance, if your baby's daily goal is eighteen ounces of milk, you're eliminating a final feeding of 3.6 ounces (one-fifth), so divide that by four:

$$3.6 \div 4 = 0.9 \text{ ounces}$$

In this case, it would be fine to round up to make the measurement easier, and to add one ounce to each of the four remaining feedings.

Now you might be wondering something: Extending the

time before the first morning feeding naturally encroaches on the next feeding of the morning just as pushing back the final feeding at night barged in on the feeding prior to it. So why do we choose to eliminate the last feeding of the night instead of the first feeding of the next morning?

The reason is simple: The bottom line is that at this point, no matter what time your baby *wakes up*, it will have been at least eight hours since the last feeding. Almost all babies will be ready to feed by then. So while the timing of the last feeding of the night is inherently a little adjustable, the first feeding of the morning is not.

Even so, you may have to adjust the second feeding of the morning, since your baby may now not be hungry by then.

For instance, if your baby had been used to waking up around 8 a.m. and feeding, and next feeding at noon, and now you've extended that wake-up feeding to 9 a.m., your baby might not take milk at noon. You may have to play that noon feeding by ear, and perhaps treat the rest of the day's feedings similarly, if there's some kind of domino effect.

We are simply recommending that, as a rule, you aim to eliminate the final feeding of the night, and play with the others, rather than eliminating the first feeding of the morning and adjusting to that.

But again, this is all up to you. We're confident you'll determine the course that is wisest for your family—for your particular situation—and act accordingly.

As long as you're giving your baby the number of calories needed for healthy weight gain and development—and not getting too nutty yourself—you and your baby should rest easy.

Naps

A common question we get from new parents is, "How many naps should my baby take per day?"

First, we should say that, in general, children don't develop their own consistent nap schedule until around six months of age. During the first two months of life, specifically, babies sleep eighteen to twenty hours a day. In the very beginning of life, the time a baby spends sleeping will be inversely proportional to age. At first, sleep will positively dominate her time. Then it will recede as she becomes able to take in more and more mental stimulation. But for the first two months or so, napping will be the norm.

If you provide your child with a routine for eating and sleeping earlier than six months, such as the Jassey Way, she may settle into a consistent nap schedule after all, but you can't be certain.

At around six months, the baby will begin to settle into her own napping routine. Here's a rough approximation of what you might expect:

At six months of age: three naps per day

One year: two naps per day

Eighteen months: Follow her cues. Generally, children this age nap once a day.

One Final Note

We realize that while we've called the Jassey Way simple, we've also thrown a lot of numbers and procedures at you. So we'd be remiss not to say that if you wish to remember nothing more than three rules, remember these:

1. Feeding a baby just because she's crying is counterproductive if you want her to sleep through the night.

2. As long as you're *increasing* the time between feedings each day—as long as you're going *forward* and not backward— you're taking a positive step toward both you and your baby getting a good night's sleep.

3. Meeting the baby's daily nutritional needs is paramount. You, the parent, can schedule and administer these feedings rather than give them "on demand."

Remember to always use—and trust in—your intuition. Give the method a chance to work. We think you'll be pleased with the results.

CHAPTER THREE

The Crying Game

Parents' Bill of Rights

Article II: Crying

1. Let's be clear: Every baby is supposed to cry at some point during the day. Most of the time, crying is a normal, healthy behavior for babies, like breathing or pooping. Babies don't necessarily have to be blissfully happy and smiley all day long. Needless to say, we're concerned if a baby doesn't regularly poop. We're just as concerned if a baby doesn't regularly cry.

2. There might be no bigger obstacle to your baby developing healthy sleep habits than an inability to cope with normal crying—your inability, that is, not your baby's.

3. The urge to feed a crying baby is strong—indescribably powerful, really. This is mostly because it's one of the more tangible steps you can take to soothe a baby, since you can't exactly talk a baby down.

4. Adults cry for many reasons, and babies cry for many reasons. In reality, healthy babies don't cry because of hunger or thirst any more than healthy adults do. So rushing to soothe a crying baby with milk is no more logical than rushing to soothe a crying adult with an intravenous drip.

5. You don't want your baby to learn to rely on feeding as a sort of pacifier. In the long run, your baby will be better off learning how to self-soothe during periods of discomfort than coming to rely on unproductive quick fixes, like the on-demand breast or bottle.

Forget What You Think You Know About Crying

The greatest arrogance of all: save the planet. What? Are these people kidding me? We haven't learned how to care for one another; we're gonna save the planet? There is nothing wrong with the planet. The planet has been through a lot worse than us. The planet isn't going anywhere. WE ARE!

—George Carlin, on environmentalists

We bring up that George Carlin quote because if you replace the environmentalists Carlin is criticizing with "parents," and you replace the planet with "babies," you get a pretty good idea of the common misunderstanding that parents have about crying: that it indicates a baby in peril or distress.

The truth is, most of the time, it's like what Carlin is saying about the earth: Your crying *baby* is going to be just fine; it's *you* who's in distress.

Dogs are going to bark, birds are going to chirp, and babies are going to cry.

Crying is their primary mode of *communication*. It's as simple as that.

To most of us, a crying baby seems like a problem—one of those problems that needs immediate solving, at that. After all, with few exceptions, it's certainly a problem when an adult cries. It seems unlikely that even the happiest baby could possibly be crying tears of joy.

To be sure, there are times when a baby *will* cry because there's a problem. We'll go over those problems later in this chapter.

But the counterintuitive reality is that there are just as many times when your baby will cry when there *isn't* a problem.

Reasonably dealing with crying is crucial to successful sleep training, whether you're using the Jassey Way or another method. (Notice how many sleep training books contain the word *cry* in the title.) But handling your crying baby in a rational, thoughtful manner will aid virtually every other facet of parenting, so even if you're not sleep training, you and your baby will benefit from a better understanding of how crying serves different functions for babies than for adults.

Crying Is Crawling

For babies, the key function of crying is to serve as their main mode of *communication*—of happy, unhappy and random thoughts alike. It might sound funny for us to point this out, but it's worth reminding ourselves while we're talking about crying: *Babies can't talk.* This is important to remember because it adds necessary context to their crying.

If you can accept that crying is a sort of primitive version of your baby's speech—instead of automatically viewing it as an expression of discomfort—then you'll be better able to react to it in a calm, sensible manner. It's fair to look at the way crying exercises the mouth and vocal cords as a sort of verbal crawling; you have to crawl before you can walk, and you have to cry before you can talk.

If your baby never cried, we'd have a lot to be concerned about, particularly in terms of neurological development. So in a way, you should be thrilled by some healthy crying. (Okay, if not thrilled, then at least a little relieved.)

If you can adopt that attitude—and we're not saying it's easy!—sleep training your baby will become much less challenging. Successful sleep training, like so many other tasks of parenting, requires careful and patient effort. If you worry that your baby is in pain every time she cries, it will be impossible to maintain that care and patience.

We need to operate from this baseline: *Crying is always communication, but it's not always a communication of pain or discomfort.*

Of course, as we've said, sometimes crying *is* an expression of discomfort or pain on the part of the baby. That's why our second baseline is: *Hunger is not the only thing that causes babies discomfort.*

(In fact, if you stick to our sleep training method, which makes sure that your baby gets the necessary number of calories per day to promote healthy weight gain and development, your baby's crying will almost *never* be an expression of hunger.)

We'll discuss the other main "cry culprits" later on in this book; for now, suffice it to say that reflexively reaching for the breast or bottle when a baby is crying is almost always misguided—both in addressing the true reason for the crying and, as we're about to go over, in relation to the baby's long-term temperament and health.

The Crying Game

Babies drive you mad . . . They get away with awful, awful things. I could see them rehearsing emotions. I snuck around the corner; I see the kid looking in the mirror, going "Ahhhh! No, no, no, no, no. AH! No, no, no. AHHHHH! Yes! That's the one!" . . . They know everything you do . . . Big head, little body.

—Robin Williams

There's a dance that almost all parents fall into with their babies, where crying is the music and milk is the finishing move. With apologies to the 1990s British psychological thriller, we call this tango the Crying Game.

Let's go over the steps.

Babies love milk—even if they're not hungry. It's like a shot of pleasure and adrenaline for them. So in addition to being a vital, life-giving source of nutrition, milk is kind of like a neonatal drug—and babies are hopeless addicts. One look at an infant's expression while feeding—eyes maybe closed, face always consumed with sucking—will confirm this.

Accordingly, it's easy to see why milk will often pacify a crying baby, at least temporarily, no matter the *reason* for the tears. If a baby is crying out of hunger, milk of course satisfies that need. If a baby is crying out of pain or discomfort, the pleasure of milk serves as a pacifying balm. Finally, if a baby is crying not because of distress, but just to communicate, as babies often do, milk might quiet the child because of its soothing, addictive quality; it's a powerful distraction.

All this is to say that regardless of what's going on inside a crying baby, milk can shift the focus. Milk can bring order to chaos. So it's no wonder most parents will instinctively reach for the breast or bottle when their infant cries.

It takes surprisingly little time for an infant to make this connection: "When I cry, I get milk." Obviously the child does not come to that conclusion *consciously*; it's instinctual, like a mouse learning to press a lever to get a piece of cheese. Since babies are little milk junkies, they like to press their lever, by crying, a lot.

And before most parents realize it, they're dancing, or playing the Crying Game:

Baby *wants* milk → Baby cries → Parents reach for milk →
Baby feeds (on unnecessary calories) → Crying stops

This would be all well and good were it not for the fact that the baby didn't *need* the milk in the first place. The baby simply *wanted* milk. The parents have, essentially, been "tricked" into feeding when it's actually counterproductive—as we're going to explain in the next section.

Think about it: How long does it take your average puppy to learn how to bark for a treat?

Don't tell us your baby isn't smarter than a puppy!

We Understand

No one likes to feel helpless. When a problem arises, we all want to find a solution—the quicker, the better. Even if we don't start searching immediately, we can't help but try to *think* of a solution. It's human nature. So no one can blame you if you fall victim to the Crying Game. You practically have to be inhuman not to.

But all parents have to remember that no one wins the Crying Game if they feed a child who does not need the milk. And that's true even if you're not structuring feedings in the name of sleep training. The bottom line is that extra calories simply carry more risk than benefit.

Following suit, parents and baby *both* win the Crying Game when Mommy and Daddy *resist* the urge to feed a crying baby only for the sake of stopping that crying. Now we'll explain why.

SAY NO TO COMFORT FOOD

Picture it. A mom criticizes her teen daughter for eating a donut after breaking up with a boyfriend. "Don't eat your feelings," she advises her.

Now picture the same mom, thirteen years earlier, giving the same child a bottle every time she cries.

A TRUE SELF-FULFILLING PROPHECY (REFLUX)

One of the ironies of automatically feeding a crying baby when it's not necessarily the right time for a feed is that too-frequent feeding may produce in your baby an abnormal amount of gas or reflux. That abnormal gas or reflux, in turn, might subject your baby to an abnormal amount of pain or discomfort. That pain or discomfort may—you guessed it—produce in your little one an abnormal amount of *crying.*

Unable or just not wanting to tolerate all this excess crying, you may be inclined to enlist the aid of that surefire cry-stopper—the bottle or breast—even more frequently. This in turn leads to more gas or reflux and more crying. And on and on it goes.

It's a pretty straightforward case of the "Band-Aid" solution actually leaving the "wound" worse off.

Stay away from that bottle Band-Aid!

THE IMPORTANCE OF SELF-SOOTHING

Another thing we like to remind our parents of is that babies are people, too. It's another principle of parenting that sounds absurd when you say it out loud, but at the same time it's disregarded by parents all the time. In this case, we're referring to the tendency to think that even though kids and adults are almost always negatively affected when they are spoiled, babies won't be. That even though learned negative behaviors are hard to undo in all of *us*, babies are a separate species immune to that susceptibility. This is not true. Babies are vulnerable to being spoiled just like the rest of us.

Since babies learn early on that crying will get an adult to feed them, and since feeding is always pleasurable to babies whether they need the milk or not, many babies will cry for milk whenever they experience some kind of discomfort—even the kinds that are normal and healthy. Who can blame them? Who wouldn't want ice cream—or some kind of other treat—when they're sad?

But, like all people, if we enable babies to get what they want whenever they want it, they'll learn nothing from these small moments of adversity. They'll start to become wired that way. They'll grow up knowing little else.

When we instead help babies learn to self-soothe, when we don't spoil them, they develop their own coping skills—skills that often last a lifetime.

We want babies to cry—because it's how they communicate and because, when it's an expression of discomfort, we don't want to interfere with a very important part of their life education.

Pick whichever analogy works best for you. Feeding a baby who doesn't need the calories is like . . . Eating ice cream while you're on a diet under the pretense that, at the moment, you're sad . . . Cheating on a test . . . Sneaking a cigarette when you supposedly have quit . . . Calling a guy or girl you said you'd never call again . . . Or come up with your own!

Make no mistake; for most of us, the urge to feed a crying baby is overwhelming. And even after they're able to resist that urge, a lot of parents can never entirely get rid of the urge itself. But with a little discipline, fortitude and persistence, you *can* keep the urge at bay for the benefit of both you and your baby. We see moms and dads achieve that victory all the time.

For more information on the link between sleeping and self-soothing, please go to Chapter 4, "What's the Big Deal About All This Anyway?"

Don't Cry It Out, Argentina

While we strictly recommend against feeding a baby just to stifle crying, we do not advocate letting babies "cry it out" without consoling them, especially during the newborn/bonding phase. There are times when you may choose to allow the baby to cry alone, providing some self-soothing practice, and other times you may choose to pick up and comfort baby as only a loving, nurturing parent can.

When you choose to console your baby, there are plenty of aids you should feel free to rely on that do not pose as much of a risk as feeding of becoming a counterproductive "crutch." These aids include:

- White noise machines/apps
- Rocking bassinets/bouncer chairs (these may come with their own noises and/or vibrations)
- Car seats

The car seat might be particularly helpful to a child who suffers from reflux; being upright may go a long way toward alleviating those symptoms.

SWADDLING (USUALLY MORE APPLICABLE AT NIGHT, BUT CAN ALSO BE EFFECTIVE DURING THE DAY)

All babies are born with a potent startle reflex, called the Moro reflex. You know when you startle in your sleep, maybe from a dream, and you wake up with, well, a start? Babies get that all the time. It can be a consistent catalyst for waking up.

For some babies, swaddling is a very effective antidote to the startle reflex; it helps them to remain asleep. Jonathan's three daughters all took to swaddling almost immediately. Lewis's two daughters, on the other hand, both seemed impervious to the intended benefit of the delicate infant-wrapping, which some parents refer to as the "baby burrito."

There are all sorts of swaddling blankets or cloths on the market. From his experience, Jonathan recommends the Miracle Blanket, which is available online and in stores. The Miracle Blanket has an extra length of Velcro strap, which wraps around the baby one and a half times, providing an extra-secure bundle that babies are less likely to wiggle out of (yes, they can have almost Houdini-like escape skills when it comes to being swaddled—even if they enjoy the comfort it provides).

Abnormal Crying and Colic

All of this talk about normal, healthy crying begs the question: What about crying that *is* a sign of something wrong?

Prolonged crying, inconsolable crying, or otherwise peculiar crying may indeed be a sign of an issue that needs to be addressed directly. In our generation, and that of our parents, grandparents, and those further and further back, that kind of crying was often referred to as colic, or the child was called a "colicky" baby. The term *colic* was so widespread even among doctors that few people ever stopped to acknowledge that it's not even a diagnosis of an illness; saying a baby has colic is in reality no more revealing than observing that a baby "cries too much."

Okay, to be fair, *baby colic* technically enjoys a *slightly* more specific definition. Kind of. Specifically, it is defined by the National Institutes of Health as "crying in a baby that lasts for longer than 3 hours a day and is not caused by a medical problem. Colic occurs in almost all babies to varying degrees. Almost all babies go through a fussy period."[1]

The truth is that it's never enough to call a baby colicky; as pediatricians, it's our job to investigate and determine *why* the baby is colicky.

We like to refer to the most common causes of colic as the "Core Four." They are gas, reflux, constipation, and milk protein allergy.

THE COLIC CORE FOUR

1. Gas

Gas can come about in one of two ways: from swallowing air while sucking on nipple or bottle or while crying; or from backed-up stools. So, needless to say, it's very normal for a baby to have gas. (Parts of Mom's diet might also contribute to gas if the child is breast-feeding.) Gas is really just air that's moving around the intestinal track. But babies sometimes have a lot of trouble handling it.

If your baby's gas appears too severe to dissolve on its own, remedies like Mylicon (generic simethicone), Mylanta, Maalox, gripe water, and glycerin suppositories can help. Make sure to follow the product's instructions for proper usage and, when possible, consult your pediatrican.

2. Gastroesophageal Reflux

When stomach contents leak back up into the esophagus, we call it gastroesophageal reflux. This is an extremely common condition in newborns and babies; a baby's esophageal sphincter—the valve muscle between the esophagus and stomach—is not fully developed, and it can sometimes send food the wrong way. Reflux can also be triggered in the first couple of months by difficulty gasping for air while eating, or struggles with burping. Some studies show that reflux can occur up to *seventy times a day* in healthy infants; it can happen so much, in fact, that most of those regurgitations go completely undetected. These are indeed, for the most part, harmless.

But some babies suffer from particularly harsh or chronic reflux, irritating the esophagus and causing the baby frequent distress. And the irritation from spitting up can be particularly severe if the baby is lying down.

If you've ever had the privilege of experiencing heartburn, you know it can be quite painful. Now imagine that feeling magnified tenfold; that's what reflux can feel like to a baby. Suffice it to say, it's more than enough to wake a sleeping infant.

If your child needs extra help soothing her reflux, there are a couple of good options.

You might first try to alleviate the gas naturally, by putting her in a car seat after feeding. Her upright position makes gravity your friend; it helps the food stay down. Any incline helps digestion, really. So you can also roll up a towel and put it under the head of the bed or couch, if she's lying down, to prop her upper body up and summon gravity that way.

If gravity doesn't prove strong enough, you can try medicines like Prevacid, Axid, Zantac and Prilosec.

Note: Some people advocate putting cereal in a baby's bottle for the final feeding to help the baby sleep through the night. We don't advocate giving a child any food whatsoever before the age of four months. (Some studies have shown that doing so triggers the production of fat cells and insulin too early, possibly leading to higher incidences of obesity and diabetes.)

The one exception to this rule is for children with very severe reflux. In these cases, thickening the feed up with a bit of cereal might be an effective antidote to the condition. The thickened feed teams with gravity to literally weigh down the child's gastroesophageal (GE) junction, which is essentially the valve between the esophagus and the stomach.

While this treatment can be effective, we strongly recommend that you consult with your pediatrician before going that route.

3. Constipation/Hard Stool

Another common gastrointestinal irritant that can cause colic is constipation—too-hard stools or total lack of evacuation.

It's worth noting here that, like adults, not all babies are "regular," as we commonly use that term. Some healthy babies "go" once a week; if such a child showed no obvious signs of distress, we would not necessarily be concerned. Other babies naturally poop frequently, and any significant constipation can cause them a lot of pain. Backed-up stools also create gas, which adds to the problem.

We find that when babies poop two to three times a day, their mood is better because they're not holding on to the poop, and the gas that's backed up with it. But again, that doesn't mean that *all* babies need to go that frequently.

To alleviate your baby's constipation, there are a range of products available to you, including Karo Syrup, medicines (like Mylanta), prune juice, glycerin suppositories, and many others.

4. Milk Protein Allergy

According to current data, 2 to 3 percent of infants suffer from an allergy to the protein in cow's milk, which is found in most commercial baby formulas.[2] Babies who breast-feed can suffer from a milk protein allergy as well, but that's said to be more rare.

In our day-to-day experience however, milk protein allergy for both formula and breast milk feeders is a bit more common than what the data shows; we see newly diagnosed cases around five to ten times every month. Many doctors might not look out for the allergy, leading to it being "underreported."

More than 95 percent of children will outgrow this allergy, but in the short term it can play havoc on a baby's system, resulting in diarrhea, frequent spitting up, vomiting, coughing, blood in the stool and, needless to say, crying.

If you suspect your baby has a milk protein allergy, contact your pediatrician, who will review with you the symptoms in question, perform a physical exam on your baby and possibly administer a stool test, to check for the presence of blood.

There are a variety of hypoallergenic formulas available for babies with milk protein allergy, including soy-based formulas; hydrolyzed formulas, in which the large protein chains are broken down into smaller, easier-to-digest chains; and amino acid–based formulas, in which the proteins are even further broken down.

DIAPER RASH

Many infants have fair and delicate skin, especially during the first couple of months of life. Fungal rashes flourish in warm, moist environments, so it's no surprise that diaper rash is not uncommon in newborns. At the same time, their skin can easily become dried out and chafed, and sometimes even bleed.

We don't recommend using diaper wipes with an infant, for this reason. Many of them have fragrances containing alcohol; even the fragrance-free wipes may contain irritants, and cause a baby further distress. If you feel you absolutely must use a wipe on your newborn under two or three months old, try to restrict it to the morning's first diaper, when there might be a particularly large specimen. After three months of age this becomes less of a risk, but wipes should still be used only sparingly, and only after your baby has passed a stool.

There are countless creams available that treat infant diaper rash effectively. These creams and gels create a barrier between the skin and the acidity that is lurking in the urine or stool.

Everyone has their favorites, including the petroleum-based creams, like A+D; Aquaphor; and the zinc oxide–based creams, like Desitin, Triple Paste, Boudreaux's Butt Paste, and Balmex.

Jonathan likes Aquaphor, but that's more from experience as a father than as a pediatrician.

ONE, SOME OR ALL OF THE ABOVE

When we get a call from a mom saying that her child is crying an abnormal amount, the first thing we do is go over the possible causes described earlier.

It's worth pointing out that this is not strictly a multiple choice question, however. An unhappy or colicky baby could be suffering not just from one of these issues, but from a combination of them, or even all of them. And parents might notice different sensitivities in their different children. Each case should be evaluated on its own, in consultation with a pediatrician.

Don't Fall into the Crying Trap

Many parents fall into the habit of feeding a crying baby because they learn early on that it often *does* stop the crying. But we don't consider that a true solution. For one thing, a true solution solves a true problem, and crying is usually *not* a true problem at all. For another thing, a solution is supposed to improve a situation—is supposed to be something "healthy"—and feeding a baby who doesn't need the milk can actually be harmful; it can compromise that baby's ability to self-soothe and, in turn, that baby's temperament, sleep habits and plenty more. In this way, feeding a crying baby is like a balm or Band-Aid, a quick fix that doesn't work toward resolving the long-term underlying issue (the need to learn self-soothing).

Don't Confuse
Correlation with Causation

Many people will claim that if a baby at least two months old starts putting her hand in her mouth a lot, it means that she's teething. But that's not true. The reality is that uniting hand and mouth is a developmental milestone that all babies will reach around two months of age, independently of teething.

This is a minor claim to "debunk," but it's a very good illustration of how, when it comes to babies, who have no voice of their own, it's all too easy to confuse correlation with causation. In other words, just because many infants reach the hand-to-mouth behavioral milestone around the same time as teething begins doesn't mean that teething *causes* that behavior.

Remember that joke about the pot roast and the grandmothers?

Automatically feeding a crying baby is like cutting off the ends of that roast. It might feel right, and it might be what your mother and her mother and her mother did, but there's no reasoning behind it.

CHEAT SHEET
How to Tell If You Should
Feed a Crying Baby

During the Day
First, answer this question: Is it time for a scheduled feeding, give or take a few minutes?

- If YES: Feed away!

- If NO: Don't feed. Soothe your baby—and help your baby learn to self-soothe—another way.

During the Night

First, answer this question: Has your baby received the daily amount of calories necessary for healthy weight gain and development?

- If YES: Don't feed. Soothe your baby—and help your baby self-soothe—another way. If your baby just won't stop crying or go to sleep and you *absolutely must* get back to sleep yourself, you may feed your baby with our blessing—as long as you stretched out this time between feedings by an additional fifteen minutes or half hour from the night before. Or, at minimum, try to make it to the time of the previous night's feeding. (If you can't go forward, at least don't go *backward*.)

- If NO: Feed away!

Did your baby receive *more* than the necessary daily amount of calories? (Did your baby overfeed?)

- If YES: Definitely don't feed now. Help your baby self-soothe another way. (At the very least, stretch out this time between feedings by an additional fifteen minutes or half hour from the night before.) And try not to overfeed tomorrow. Remember, you are training your baby's stomach to align with your baby's mind and ability to sleep through the night. When you overfeed, you run the risk of throwing that training out of whack, of causing reflux issues, or even of causing excessive weight gain.

Did your baby receive *less* than the necessary daily amount of calories? (Did your baby not feed enough?)

- If YES: Feed now! And please get back on track tomorrow by sticking to a reliable feeding schedule that gives your baby the necessary daily amount of calories and helps stretch out your baby's stomach to enable consistent, healthy sleep habits.

In this regard, the Jassey Way is flexible, deferring to your parental instincts and judgment to decide when crying is okay, and when enough is enough.

CHAPTER FOUR

What's the Big Deal About All This Anyway?

The Immutable Importance of Sleep— for Both Family and Baby

Parents' Bill of Rights

Article III: Sleep

1. Sleep is not something human beings can afford to "catch" when their time allows for it. Like eating well, and engaging in a certain degree of physical and mental activity, getting good, consistent sleep is something humans *need* to be healthy. Its restorative powers are simply irreplaceable.

2. Human parents don't stop being human when they become parents (see #1). To be a good human parent, you need some good human sleep!

3. Babies, even tiny infants, are also human. The healthier your baby's sleep behavior is, the healthier your child will be overall.

4. Babies don't "naturally" hurt their parents' sex lives; that would serve no evolutionary purpose! It's parents' own behavior *around* babies that has the potential to seriously disrupt the intimacy they previously enjoyed.

5. A new baby might inevitably throw a wrench into the emotions of her siblings. That problem will only be compounded if the infant is not sleeping well, and thusly monopolizing her parents' attention and energy.

When their little one keeps them up at all hours, parents feel, among other things, like they're going out of their minds.

Of course, this temporary insanity is such a widespread symptom of new parenthood that, as we've said, many people have come to believe it's a necessary part of parenthood, like changing diapers or reading *Goodnight Moon.*

As we've also said, it is *not* at all necessary.

But in this chapter, we'd like to impress upon you the fact that sleeplessness is not only unnecessary for new parents; it can be downright dangerous. We might even go so far as to say that being *well rested* is what's *necessary* in properly caring for a newborn.

Sure, most people don't need to be convinced of the value of a good night's sleep, but not *all* of its benefits are completely obvious—especially when it comes to looking after an infant.

So in this chapter, we'll try to drive home the harmful effects of a lack of sleep on people in general, and families with a new-born in particular.

And if all that's not convincing enough, we'll also explore the reasons that sleep training is so incredibly important for the health and well-being of the baby, too.

Sleep Deprivation: The Dangers for Us All

We all know what can happen when we don't get enough sleep; we can become irritable, sluggish, depressed, paranoid, even hallucinatory. We risk becoming zombie-like shells of our true selves—zombies without that signature unlimited zombie energy, that is.

What's truly scary, however, is the possibility that, just as in a classic horror movie, many of us are *already* those zombies, and we don't even know it.

At least, that was the message that came out of a major study conducted by the Gallup organization in December of 2013.

That study found that 40 percent of Americans currently get fewer than the seven hours of sleep per night generally accepted as the minimum necessary to maintain optimal health. The average amount of nightly sleep per person in this country was discovered to be only 6.8 hours.[1]

Kind of makes you wonder how much better things would be if our national average *did* meet the minimum!

Certainly none of this will come as very surprising news to you, but if you're about to have—or already have—a newborn, it's probably somewhat alarming news. Because never, in the history of the world, has anyone ever told a new parent: "Finally you'll have an opportunity to catch up on all that sleep you've been missing."

So sleep training is important for many new parents not only because being well rested is important for *parenting*, but because they would do well to get some consistently good sleep just for *living*.

In fact, studies reveal additional dangers of insufficient sleep seemingly all the time. Recently, the Huffington Post published an article concisely summarizing the conclusions of the most current research on sleep deprivation:[2]

Only One Night of Insufficient Sleep Can Lead to an Increase in Your

- Hunger

- Vulnerability to having an accident

- Skin aging

- Vulnerability to catching a cold

- Emotional volatility

While One Night of Insufficient Sleep Can Lead to a Decrease in Your

- Brain tissue

- Attractiveness to others

- Ability to focus

- Memory

A Chronic Lack of Sleep Can Lead to an
Increase *in the Risk of*

- Stroke

- Obesity

- Some cancers

- Diabetes

- Heart disease

And a **Decrease** *in*

- Sperm count

Sleep Deprivation: The Dangers for New Parents

You don't need drugs when you have a kid. You're awake,
you're paranoid, you smell bad; it's the same thing.

—Robin Williams

Now that we've reviewed how destructive sleep deprivation is in its own right, let's take a look at the particular dangers that come with sleep deprivation when it plagues a family with a newborn.

Make no mistake: Sleep deprivation is a family affair, a "global" issue. As with any illness, no one family member can suffer in isolation; the deprived individual's symptoms will likely affect his or her behavior, and thusly have a ripple effect on everyone else in the house to some extent.

THE SAFETY OF THE BABY

Babies are a lot to care for even on one's best day. If you're tired too much of the time, your ability to provide your child with a safe home environment, and to protect her from any external threats, becomes severely compromised.

We've heard horror stories of moms falling asleep while nursing in a chair, and being woken up by the sound of the child hitting the floor.

Those incidents are very rare, and we don't mean to scare you. But we do want to make an impression; let's leave it at that.

BABY BLUES

The cause or causes of postpartum depression have not been totally established. It seems likely that hormones have something to do with it, but while all new moms experience hormone fluctuation and withdrawal, all new moms do not suffer from postpartum depression (PPD), so the scientific community is not yet certain of the connection.

We can be certain, however, that any mom who *does* suffer from PPD, at any intensity, is not going to *benefit* from being tired all the time. And of course, the mom who does *not* suffer from PPD would not want to risk her good fortune by weakening her system with fatigue.

Mom is the nucleus of the family; this fact can be obscured with an infant present, since the baby naturally commands so much attention from everyone. But the reality is that Mom is the center, and family life flows through her. If she is unhappy from a lack of sleep, or even if she's just "not her best" or a little "run-down," this will affect not only her ability to bond with the baby, but also the spirit of the proud new dad and any siblings.

In other words, Mom will ideally be a bright sun, full of energy, around which the rest of the family orbits; she should not be a black hole of fatigue and lethargy, into which the rest of the family slides.

DESPONDENT DAD

Needless to say, we can say much of the same for Dad as well.

STEWING SIBLINGS

Siblings of a newborn sometimes have a difficult time adjusting emotionally to the addition of an infant to the family, and the attendant parental attention that comes with the baby. To a young child who doesn't fully understand it all, the change in the air of the household might seem like a total parental eclipse.

This can be an inevitable symptom of bringing a new baby home, but while it might be unavoidable, it can at least be minimized. But if that infant is not getting any sleep, and sapping all her parents' energy and time as a result, her presence will wear on the spirits and emotions of her siblings all the more.

ENJOYING YOUR BABY

This lethargy is not just damaging because it wears on the psyches of the family; it's also unfortunate because it does this at *the exact same time* when everyone should be feeling uplifted.

There's *taking care* of a baby, and then there's *enjoying a baby*, and the latter is one of the reasons many of us have one in the first place. Yet while there is limitless information available on the *taking care* part, the resources trumpeting the *enjoyment* of the experience are few and far between.

But what most moms and dads discover very early on in the journey of parenthood is that, unfortunately, taking care of a baby often does interfere with enjoying her at the same time. And this is never more true than when caring for your baby prevents you from getting consistently good sleep yourself.

Think about how different life is when you're exhausted. The all-nighters you pulled in college to study for an exam or to complete a project. The times in your twenties when you'd stay out all night and still go to work the next day. The nights when, for whatever reason, you just couldn't fall asleep. Think about how terrible it usually was the next day. How, no matter what you were doing, you couldn't really appreciate it or enjoy it—or be very good at doing it, if it was something that needed doing—because you weren't really present. You were a sleepless zombie. Lights on, nobody's home.

If you're going to be, or currently are, a first-time parent, those memories of exhaustion might be a fair approximation of what to expect from caring for an infant who sleeps erratically. If you've already raised a baby, you may even be thinking that in reality, it's much worse than that. And it goes on for a much longer time.

The point is that you need your sleep to be on your game not only when it comes to the *taking care* part of parenting, but for the *enjoyment* part of parenting as well.

LET'S TALK ABOUT SEX

Yet another great irony of raising a child is that it has the potential to kill the very same innate drive that led to that child's creation in the first place. This has been so pervasive among parents for so long that it's well past the point of cliché. It seems almost to be an accepted fact of parenting life. But it doesn't have to be.

Fatigue is doubtlessly the number one culprit when new parents' sex lives lose their magic. It's like what we said in the last section; if you're exhausted for long enough, you have a tough time enjoying *anything*. All you want to do is sleep. The idea of doing anything strenuous or energetic—and doing it in a place that would be comfortable for *sleeping* no less!—begins to seem downright idiotic.

At the same time, since you're energy-sapped all the time, it's harder to attend to your physical appearance, and you might naturally begin to feel less attractive, which only compounds the problem.

WEAKENED IMMUNITY

Imagine a family where the immunity of Mom and Dad and the kids is compromised from fatigue as a result of taking care of a tiny infant whose immune system is fairly weak in the first place—it's a veritable powder keg for illness. Colds, flu, other types of infections—these are bad enough under normal circumstances, but when a baby is involved, the consequences can be much higher. So it's not hard to see why it's especially important for families with newborns to get a decent amount of shut-eye for the sake of everyone's health.

Sleep Deprivation: The Dangers for Babies

....

I know people today who are in their thirties, and I can tell they were the kind of babies whose parents never said no to them.

—Andrew H., father of two

SELF-SOOTHING

We know we're repeating ourselves. It's only because, when it comes to babies, if something's actually worth saying, it usually is worth saying a hundred times. And one of those things is that it's so important for your baby to learn how to self-soothe.

As a culture, we have collectively gotten used to instant gratification. Almost everything is now "on demand." If you want to reach someone, you call that person's cell phone; everyone is theoretically available all the time. (If people can't *talk* at the moment, at least they usually can text.) And if you want an answer to a question, forget looking it up in some book; there's Google. Heck, we don't even have to wait to have our photographs developed anymore; even a Polaroid is a dinosaur compared to a digital camera. And when was the last time you found yourself waiting for *mail* and not an *email*?

We're not philosophers or psychiatrists—at least, not "officially"—and we don't want to be looked at as the old men screaming, "You kids get off my lawn!"

But we can't help but feel that as we more and more become an instant gratification, on-demand society, fewer of us will be able to practice the important skills of patience and thoughtfulness as individuals. We fear that we'll no longer be able to tolerate delayed gratification. And this concern is strong enough already; who knows how dire things might get with the new generations coming up, the children who know their way around an iPad before they can speak a single word.

So while there is no doubt that the ability to self-soothe has been an essential human skill for as long as the human race has existed, we can't help but feel that it's more important now than ever.

In our eyes, feeding a crying baby in the middle of the night to get her to go back to sleep is robbing her of the opportunity to learn some valuable life skills. Instead of working toward instilling in her the value of patience and the ability to soothe herself, without help from outside forces, you are giving her a taste of our on-demand culture even *before* she can get a hand on an iPad. You are conditioning her to *expect* instant gratification.

Hopefully she'll grow out of that; she'll mature. But what if she doesn't?

Now you might be thinking, "Does it really matter how we 'condition' such a tiny baby? Will things we teach her now *really* show up later in life?"

In response, we'd ask you to consider how much our understanding of human development has evolved over time, and especially in recent years. It seems as if every week brings a new study showing how adult behavior and traits are shaped by experiences in childhood. And the age when this shaping is said to begin keeps getting lower and lower, not higher.

At the same time, we're constantly discovering new ways in which genetics shape our development.

It's hard to imagine that we'll ever know how much of who we are is determined by nature and how much by nurture.

But at this point, it's impossible not to conclude that our entire lives are in play. That there's nothing that happens to us at *any time* in our lives that doesn't have at least the potential to affect us in the long run.

With that understanding in mind, we are confident that yes, the things we teach babies—even infants—do have the power to influence who they become as adults.

TEMPER, TEMPER, TEMPER

All parents fear the so-called terrible twos, and that period is, to some extent, unavoidable. But one misconception is that your little one will be sung "Happy Birthday" at her second birthday party and then, all of a sudden, lose the ability to control herself.

The reality is that while it is true that certain physiological changes take place within a child as she gets older, it is also true that positively managing the child's behavior must begin long before then.

This is particularly important when it comes to self-soothing, because the ability to endure delayed gratification goes hand-in-hand with a person's temperament.

Think about it. When we describe people as spoiled, we usually mean that they can't handle not getting what they want when they want it. Delayed gratification irritates, angers or upsets them—or all three.

We all know people like this. We can't conclude that *all* of them were fed on demand as babies, but, like Andrew H., the dad we quote earlier, we definitely have our suspicions.

In this way, scheduled feedings, scheduled sleep, delayed gratification and learning to self-soothe might not *guarantee* that a child grows up to possess a healthy temperament, but *not* allowing the child to develop those skills can only *harm* the likelihood of it.

You might think of temperament as an invisible tree growing inside your child, a tree that will live inside her her whole life. When your child is a baby, that tree is just a sapling. If you water it correctly, it stands a good chance of growing up healthy and strong and tall. If you do not, it may grow to be brittle and barren.

The ability to self-soothe is the seed of that tree.

The baby is the template of the adult.

Co-Sleeping

As we've said time and again, we accept that there are so many ways to raise a healthy baby that to criticize any parenting method that's carried out by thoughtful and well-meaning parents is often unfair and perhaps naïve. Still, there is one practice that's become widely accepted that we strongly recommend *against*: co-sleeping, or sharing your bed with your baby. (An exception would be short-term extenuating circumstances, but even those should be kept to a minimum.)

SAFETY

During medical school and pediatric residency, every doctor hears a few co-sleeping horror stories. You hear about sound-sleeping parents who accidentally roll over onto their child during the night, suffocating her. You hear about infants falling off the bed themselves and fracturing an extremity in the process or, in severe cases, dying. Or newborns unwittingly pushed out of bed by sleeping parents, with the same terrible results.

Finally, one of the hidden dangers of co-sleeping lies in the fact that a bed made for adults is simply not designed for the bodies of babies. This risk can manifest itself in any number of ways (we described a couple of them above), but one of the more tragic relevant stories Jonathan heard during his training was of a child who somehow wormed his way into getting his head stuck between the headboard and mattress of his parents' bed and died from resulting injuries.

Are these cases extreme? Yes. Are they rare? Yes. Could these hypotheticals even be called alarmist? Perhaps.

But we bring them up for a good reason. The bottom line is that co-sleeping is so *unnecessary* that we don't see any value in assuming the risk, as low as it may be, in the first place. Why tempt fate when there's no real benefit in doing so?

It's true that, as with anything else involving babies, there are some studies that show supposed benefits to babies from co-sleeping, but these are all a little obscure and, to put it simply, not commonly accepted.

Let's be real. Co-sleeping is all about the parents' desires or needs. It's a way for parents who never want to leave their child's side to accomplish just that.

We are inherently suspicious of any parenting technique that is so obviously weighted to the parents' wants over the potential benefits to the child. To us, this practice seems all risk and no payoff. But the physical risk of co-sleeping is not the only risk we see.

DEVELOPMENTAL RISKS

In the last section, we talked about the real, if low, risk of physically smothering or otherwise injuring a child while co-sleeping. But there's another kind of smothering parents should be wary of: emotional smothering.

We talk a lot about the need for babies to learn the ever-valuable skill of self-soothing. But if Mommy and Daddy are so close to baby during the night—the very time when learning to sleep, the foundation of self-soothing, is so important—then how can the baby accomplish it? Mommy and Daddy are like ever-present crutches in that respect.

And this is before we get to the key question: When will it *end*?

When will you decide that it's time for your child to finally sleep on her own? One year? Two years? No matter when you decide that *that* transition should take place, it promises to be somewhat difficult because the child will be so acclimated to being next to you while she sleeps.

For the sake of healthy emotional development, a child should learn to rely on her *own* space as safe and comforting. This is easier for a child when she's an infant; never knowing anything different, she naturally "grows into it," so to speak. But an older child who has grown into a completely opposite setting—who is consciously used to sleeping next to Mommy and Daddy—might have a tough time leaving that safe haven, and sleeping by herself, when the time comes.

In fact, we've heard many cautionary tales about co-sleeping over the years that invariably include parents deciding that it was time for the co-sleeping with their infant or toddler to come to an end, only to have the child become hysterical when left to sleeping in her own room. And why wouldn't she? If she wants to remain in the bed with Mommy and Daddy, she might do whatever it takes to achieve that return to her parents' bed. There's no doubt that if you ask enough parents who have tried co-sleeping, you'll hear a fair share of these stories.

The bottom line is that setting emotional and physical boundaries for your children is a hugely important part of parenting. It's necessary for the healthy psychological development of the child. Co-sleeping violates that principle in a fundamental way.

A married couple we know recently got divorced, which led to their four-year-old daughter learning to sleep in her bed alone for the first time. Her parents had only intended to co-sleep for several months, but months had rolled into a year and a year had rolled into multiple years. There was never a good time to make the transition. Finally they were forced into it due to the circumstances of their separation. Had that unfortunate event not occurred, who knows when the transition would have happened?

INTIMACY

We talked about this earlier, but it certainly is worth repeating here. When taking care of a baby begins to dominate a couple's life—when it begins to become the focal point of their life together, rather than a happy complement to it—they run the risk of losing some of the intimacy they share. Simply put, taking care of a baby is a miracle, but it's not always the biggest turn-on. After a child is born, a couple eventually still has to find their way back to normal intimacy if they don't want to sacrifice their romantic life together. Co-sleeping makes that challenge that much harder.

Parenting Irony Alert

Think about it this way. It's a cliché that kids can "get between" their parents when it comes to their sex lives. But when we say that, we of course mean it figuratively. But parents who have their baby share their bed with them are *literally* putting a child between them. It's not hard to imagine the negative consequences of that.

CLOSE SLEEPING

While we don't recommend co-sleeping, we are in favor of what we call "close sleeping"—that is, sleeping in the same room as your infant, but not in the same bed. We advise that parents "close sleep" until their baby is getting around seven or eight hours of uninterrupted sleep on a consistent basis. This way, if you do have to wake up during the night to soothe an upset baby, you won't have to go far.

Obviously we don't mean taking a sleeping bag into the nursery and sleeping on the floor next to your baby's crib—unless you're a big fan of camping. For most parents, "close sleeping" will mean keeping the child's bassinet near their bed, so they can rock her back to sleep without being fully awake themselves.

CHAPTER FIVE

Of Breast and Bottle

Parents' Bill of Rights

Article IV: Breast and Formula Feeding

1. No matter which approach you choose—breast-feeding or formula feeding—you are being a good mother. Either way, you are providing your baby with the nutrients needed for healthy weight gain and development.

2. The great breast-feeding debate has spiraled out of control. In reality, it's a matter of orange juice versus apple juice. It's not orange juice versus antifreeze.

3. Nutritionally, breast milk and formula are essentially equally healthy for babies, with breast milk carrying a very slight edge.

4. The need for a good, consistent feed supersedes the question of breast or formula—even forgetting the issue of sleep training.

5. But on the subject of sleep training: A baby that "grazes" rather than taking substantial, consistent feeds might have trouble sleeping consistently.

6. The real advantage of breast-feeding is the special bonding that it can foster. If it proves to be more of a struggle—physically or mentally—breast-feeding is probably not worth its presumed slight nutritional advantage.

7. In this area of parenting, we are *pro-mommy-and-daddy-situational. We support whichever choice you make.* Each approach has advantages and disadvantages, and we'll go over them in a bit. (Cards on the table: Our five daughters were all formula fed.)

8. In parenting, you have to "pick your battles." For some moms, breast-feeding will come easily, or easily enough, and it will be yet another priceless part of motherhood. For others, it might be more of a battle. Only Mom can decide if it's a battle worth picking. No one else can do this for her.

9. No mom should be pressured into choosing one approach over the other, and no mom should be criticized for choosing one approach over the other.

10. Both breast-feeding and formula feeding work in tandem with the Jassey Way of sleep training.

A Personal Choice

When a new mom asks, "Should I breast-feed or bottle feed?" the answer should always be "Yes!" In other words, both of those options are just fine with us, and will be just fine for your baby.

To be sure, among other organizations, the American Academy of Pediatrics (AAP), the American Medical Association (AMA), the American Dietetic Association (ADA) and the World Health Organization (WHO) endorse breast-feeding as the ideal way of feeding babies—mostly due to the slight nutritional advantages it's reputed to have.[1] But it's important for parents to remember that that's an ideal, just as five servings of fruits and vegetables per day, or eight glasses of water, or seven hours of sleep are ideals for adults. For many of us, achieving those ideals on a daily basis would necessarily compromise other parts of our lives. So we look at those ideals in a big-picture context, and we adjust accordingly. We do our best. Most of us do not eat five servings of fruits and veggies every day, but we are nonetheless able to achieve good health. And it's the same with breast-feeding. With all due respect to our colleagues and moms everywhere, the plain truth is that we've never observed a difference in health between formula-fed children and children raised on breast milk. We're not discounting that there might be a real difference between these two versions of milk. But we haven't seen it.

As we'll say time and again—because it's worth repeating—Mom must look at the breast-feeding versus formula feeding choice in a similarly global manner. As long as your baby gets the amount of milk necessary per day for healthy weight gain and development—preferably in consistent, comfortably spaced feedings—it doesn't matter if that milk is from the breast or if it's formula.

As we said before, we're pro-mommy-and-daddy-situational here. We recommend to the parents we guide that they make their own big-picture decision based on the ease or challenges Mom experiences in breast-feeding, and on the context of the rest of their lives.

As pediatricians, we have two main goals—that your baby is healthy and happy, and that you, the parents, are healthy and happy.

So in one respect, we "agree" with the AAP, AMA and other organizations that recommend breast-feeding; for many parents, this way of feeding facilitates health and happiness on the part of baby and Mom and Dad.

But for other parents, while breast-feeding might cover our "health" goal, it may to some extent undo the "happy" goal. For those parents, we'd recommend formula feeding.

Make no mistake—you, as parents, should be happy. Every day with your baby should be a joy. Of course, there are limitless chores, pains and frustrations folded into that joy; those are un-avoidable. But if those little tribulations *overtake* the joy of par-enting your baby, we have a problem.

Incidentally, we don't say that parenting should be a joy *only* because we want you to be happy. We also say it because, to put it plainly, happy parents make better parents. So our in-voking of joy is a clinical recommendation as much as it is a "friendly" one.

Breast and Bottle and Formula

In our practice, when we talk about breast or bottle feeding (we prefer "or" to "versus"), we generally mean breast milk or baby formula. But of course there is a third approach, which is pumping breast milk and then feeding that milk *via* the bottle. This chapter will deal mainly with breast milk and formula.

Remain Calm

When it comes to the breast or bottle question, we're hard-pressed to come up with other debates that inspire as much passion, obstinacy and, sadly, hostility and passive aggression.

There are breast-feeding moms who look at formula-feeding moms as if, by formula feeding, they're giving their babies a diet of Pinot and cigarettes. There are formula-feeding moms who view breast-feeding moms as zealous, vaccine-eschewing hippies. Both of these stereotypes are totally off-base.

As we said before, both breast milk and formula are perfectly healthy for babies, so this debate really only serves to bring unnecessary pressure and criticism on innocent moms. It's one of the most regrettable developments in baby culture that we've seen in our time practicing pediatrics.

A Levelheaded Approach

We understand that the decision whether to breast-feed or bottle feed is a very personal one and that, ultimately, it will be based primarily on information you collect outside of these pages, whether from your doctor, other books, your family, your friends or other sources.

We would not try to steer you in one direction over the other. Just as science does not, in reality, indicate that one approach is unquestionably best, we have no experience from practicing pediatrics that forcefully points to one over the other.

At the same time, we'd be remiss not to make sure that when you're considering this important decision, you are framing the three options in the clearest light.

So first let's go over the salient pros and cons of each method in summary; afterward, we'll discuss these factors in detail, so that you can make the decision that's best for you and your baby.

All Things Considered

....

*Breast-feeding is nice, but it's just one piece
of the puzzle. You're probably better off bottle feeding
in Tahiti than you are breast-feeding in a stressful
environment like New York City.*

—Geri B., mother of two

BREAST-FEEDING

Pros
Nutrition: Many studies show that breast milk is nutritionally superior to formula (we'll summarize the established benefits in the next section). Furthermore, the composition

of breast milk changes with the nutritional needs of your growing baby.

Bonding: As we said before, breast-feeding, ideally, offers an intimacy between Mom and baby that can't be replicated any other way.

Cost: Unless you have an uncle who works at Similac or one of the other manufacturers, breast-feeding is inherently cheaper than formula feeding, for obvious reasons.

Health benefits to Mom: Breast-feeding releases the hormone oxytocin into Mom's system. This helps her heal in various ways after delivery (reducing the size of the uterus, reducing bleeding and enhancing mood). Some studies have shown a possible association between breast-feeding and reduced rates of breast and ovarian cancer, along with other diseases, down the road.

(Shortly, we'll explain why we find the proven nutritional benefits of breast milk to the baby to be somewhat slight; we consider the benefits to Mom to be similarly marginal.)

Cons

Imprecise: Mom can pump milk when her breast is full, and gauge the volume using a measuring cup. But it goes without saying that this baseline will naturally fluctuate, due to the baby's changing appetite and other factors. Since the Jassey Way depends on the direct relationship between feeding and sleeping, these fluctuations make it ever so slightly more difficult to implement. (But this is by no means a deal breaker!)

Delayed sleep training: Since it generally takes a few days of pumping and feeding for Mom to kick-start that engine and get consistent milk in, breast-feeding inherently delays any sleep training. (Again, not a deal breaker.)

Potential discomforts and difficulties: For many women, breast-feeding does not "take" right away. It can be painful, frustrating and a source of stress for Mom (and therefore also for baby).

Dad can't breast-feed.

BOTTLE FEEDING WITH BREAST MILK

Pros
Precision/convenience and nutrition: The nutritional benefits of breast milk with the precision and convenience of bottle feeding.

Dad can feed, too.

Con
Lacks the bonding experience of breast-feeding: The nutritional benefits of breast milk *without* the Mommy-baby bonding experience that is the heart of breast-feeding.

Needless to say, breast milk has the same nutritional parameters whether it's fed to your baby via breast or bottle. These two approaches differ slightly in the context of the Jassey Way, as we discussed in Chapter 2.

Aside from that initial difference, we look at them as the same. So for the rest of *this* chapter, unless otherwise noted, we'll use the term *breast-feeding* to mean breast milk, whether fed by breast or bottle, and *formula feeding* to mean just that.

FORMULA FEEDING

Pros

Precision: It's easy to keep track of baby's exact consumption when you're working with formula.

Convenience: You can feed with very little notice, as long as you have formula on hand.

Sleep training: Makes the Jassey Way—almost any sleep training, in our estimation—a bit easier.

Dad can feed, too: Not only can Dad get in on the bonding action, but Dad being able to feed the baby will likely help Mom's bonding as well. If Mom is solely responsible for feeding baby all the time—without any mental break from that responsibility—it may wear on her, and even negatively affect her body language while feeding—something the baby might tacitly pick up on. But if Dad can occasionally provide Mom with a respite from the job, she might feel like her feedings are less of an *obligation* and, as a result, more enjoyable on the whole.

Cons

Nutritional disadvantage: It's slight—and in our eyes even that slight advantage is only *presumed*—but when it comes to your baby, that still might be convincing enough. And that is fine with us!

Lack of deeper bonding: Feeding your baby with a bottle is still one of the more magical experiences you'll experience in life. But it's obviously not quite the same as breast-feeding.

Note on Bonding: Make no mistake: If you formula feed your baby, you're going to experience a special bonding with the child all the same. And Dad's going to experience it, too. So we're not saying that breast-feeding *necessarily* fosters a more special bonding experience, only that some moms might feel that way, and we completely respect that.

Note on Caffeine and Breast-Feeding: Many moms ask us if it's unwise to drink coffee or other caffeinated beverages if they are breast-feeding their baby. In short, we wouldn't worry about it; we've never observed a baby who was "wired" because her mom had been drinking a lot of caffeine. We'd advise sticking to the morning or early afternoon when consuming caffeinated beverages, just to make extra sure they don't affect your baby's sleep. But you certainly don't need to "pump and dump" breast milk that may have a bit of caffeine in it, as you would with an alcoholic beverage.

Note on Nipple Confusion: In the early weeks of life, it's possible for a bottle-fed baby to "forget" how to breast-feed, because the mouth motions required are different. In practice, we don't see babies who have been accustomed to breast-feeding having trouble going back to the breast after some bottle feeding, but we do occasionally see the inverse: babies who are used to the breast having trouble with the *bottle*. This is not such an epidemic that all breast-feeding moms should be wary of it. We would simply advise moms who breast-feed to mix a bottle in *once in a while* to combat any risk of nipple confusion.

Proven Benefits of Breast-Feeding

We can't just say breast milk is only slightly superior to standard baby formula (Similac, Enfamil, etc.) without explaining ourselves.

First off, in our more than thirty years of practicing pediatrics, we've never observed any correlation between the health of our patients and whether they were breast- or formula-fed. And it's literally our job to notice such things.

But it goes without saying that you don't need to take our word for it. You can do your own research. What you're bound to find is that as of our writing this book, there hasn't been any study that showed that breast-feeding significantly *protected against* any common illness. Breast-feeding has only been proven to *reduce the already small risk of* a limited number of conditions that are themselves uncommon, and many of which are linked to genetic factors in the first place.

For instance, take what might be the most attention-grabbing result in the following list: SIDS. One study showed that breast-feeding was linked to a 50 percent reduction in the risk of SIDS. But the rate of SIDS in the United States is already microscopic: fewer than one death for every one thousand births (less than 0.1 percent). And this study is not even saying that breast-feeding alone is linked to reducing *that* number by half; rather, it shows that *along with other factors*, breast-feeding might work to halve that number.

In most of these cases, the result is tantamount to saying "you have a reduced chance of being struck by lightning over here than you do over there."

It's undeniably true, but it's not necessarily compelling.

Again, it comes down to a personal choice.

THE "HARD" EVIDENCE

In 2007, the National Center for Biotechnology Information published a paper called "Breast-feeding and Maternal and Infant Health Outcomes in Developed Countries," which summarized the "evidence on the effects of breast-feeding on short- and long-term infant and maternal health outcomes in developed countries."[2]

In English: The authors reviewed all of the legitimate studies on breast-feeding and long-term health that were out there, and judged all the data.

The website PhDinParenting.com summarized the study's findings in one list, which includes the following highlights.[3]

It's now been more than six years since the meta-analysis was published, but this evidence, culled from multiple studies, remains relevant today.

Among other findings, compared to babies who were not breast-fed, babies who were breast-fed were found to have:

- *Fewer ear infections*: 23 percent lower incidence

- *Fewer cases of nonspecific gastroenteritis*: 64 percent less risk

- *Less risk of asthma*: 27 percent less risk for those with no family history, and 40 percent less risk for those with a family history of asthma

- *Less risk of childhood leukemia*: 19 percent less risk of acute lymphocytic leukemia, and 15 percent less risk of acute myelogenous leukemia

- *Less risk of sudden infant death syndrome (SIDS)*: 36 percent less risk. A later study found a 50 percent reduction in risk. (The rate of SIDS is fewer than one death for every one thousand births to begin with, so both the risk and the reduction are small.)

The meta-analysis took into account a range of factors including, in some cases, the age of the babies studied and how long they were breast-fed.

Some of the additional findings not listed above relate to conditions diagnosed later in life, such as diabetes (Type 1 and Type 2), some of which were less conclusive.

The research and analysis are widely available and worth consideration. In the end, the decision to breast-feed is and should be a personal choice, and one that in a perfect world would not cause undue stress, guilt or judgment. It comes down to what you feel is best for you and your baby.

DINNER AND THE DAILY NEWSPAPER

To better understand what we mean by taking a big-picture perspective on the breast-feeding and formula-feeding decision, bear with us for a little analogy.

Chefs and daily newspaper editors—what's left of them—will tell you that a dinner is like a newspaper in the following way: You can spend as much time as you want getting each one perfect, but if you don't get each one out *on time*, it may as well be a failure—no matter how "good" it is.

Breast-feeding is similar. If, in practice, breast-feeding results in feeding your baby at erratic times, or if it means Mom is stressed out from it due to physical discomfort or fatigue, or if it has any other destructive consequences, then it doesn't matter how "good" breast milk itself is or how good for the baby breast-feeding is supposed to be; as with a dinner that's perfect but two hours late, or a morning paper that hits newsstands at 3 p.m., the extra time and effort put into it is usually not worth it.

COLOSTRUM

At the end of pregnancy, and through the first few days after birth, the breasts of mammals—including Mom's—produce colostrum: a yellow-ish, almost butterscotch milk, thick and sticky. Colostrum is low in volume but high in carbohydrates, protein and antibodies, and also acts as a laxative, easing the passage of baby's first stools. For these reasons, it is often called "liquid gold" or "high-octane milk." The breasts transition from colostrum to milk during the first two weeks after birth; if Mom is feeding early and often, mature milk may come in after only a few days.[4]

Breast-feeding moms will naturally feed their babies colostrum in the first days of life as a matter of course.

But some moms who ultimately intend to formula feed might

choose to breast-feed for the first few weeks of life in order to take advantage of the added benefits of the colostrum.

Again, it's a personal choice. If Mom wants to delay formula to make sure baby gets all of the colostrum, that's great. If Mom wants to begin formula feeding immediately, for the sake of sleep training or for other reasons, that's great, too.

CHAPTER SIX

Tooth Eruption, Sleep Disruption and Resetting the Clock

Tooth Eruption

Tooth eruption is not the emo band that used to open for Pavement in the nineties. It's the technical term used to describe the process of teeth sprouting through the gums and becoming visible in the mouth.

In babies, when the very first teeth erupt, this is called the primary dentition stage or, more commonly, *teething*.

We mention the term *tooth eruption* because it's much more descriptive than *teething* of what the baby is likely going through. *Teething* sounds like a dainty process whereby little teeth politely ask for permission to come in, take off their hats after they show up, and sit quietly. *Tooth eruption* is closer to what it must feel like; like what an adult goes through when a troublesome wisdom tooth fights its way to the surface. Tooth eruption is what babies would call it if they could describe it to us.

The first eruption, the teething, can begin as early as three months of age, but usually starts around six to ten months, with the appearance of the lower central incisors: the two bottom front teeth. Then come the top four front; then the rest fill in slowly, usually in pairs—one on the top, one on the bottom—fanning out from the central incisors. Here's what to expect, generally:

Upper Teeth

Central incisors come in at 6 to 12 months.

Lateral incisors come in at 9 to 13 months.

Canines come in at 16 to 22 months.

First molars come in at 12 to 18 months.

Second molars come in at 24 to 33 months.

Lower Teeth

Central incisors come in at 6 to 12 months.

Lateral incisors come in at 10 to 16 months.

Canines come in at 17 to 23 months.

First molars come in at 12 to 18 months.

Second molars come in at 24 to 33 months.

Here are some other rough guidelines to keep in mind:

- Every six months, around four teeth come in.

- Girls usually experience tooth eruption a bit earlier than boys.

- Lower teeth usually come in before upper teeth.

- Teeth usually come in in pairs—one on the right, one on the left.

- Primary teeth ("baby teeth") usually all come in by the time a child is two or three years old.

As you can see, teething is a lengthy process, not fully culminating until two to three years of age. But for our purposes right now, what you need to know is that the eruption might be very painful for your child from the time it begins, around six to nine months of age (or possibly even earlier) until around two to three years of age. Thank God we don't remember teething later on in life.

SLEEP DISRUPTION

By now it should go without saying that this little gum excavation may interfere with your baby's sleep behavior, no matter how well conditioned it has been. (Additional events that might interfere include vacations, illnesses, and other major environmental changes or disturbances.)

Teething is therefore perhaps the first major test of your child's ability to cope with significant distress and to self-soothe. To add to the stakes, the inflammation from teething seems to be worse at night.

Resetting the Clock

If your baby's normal sleep cycle has been upset for more than three consecutive days and nights—as may well happen with teething—it's probably necessary to "reset the clock"—that is, to get your child's circadian rhythm back on track with the help of external measures.

BEWARE THE RETURN OF THE BOTTLE

We've seen babies who were great sleepers suddenly become poor ones in the wake of teething or another trauma—but not on account of the trauma alone. In these cases, the parents fell into a tempting but very dangerous trap. Since, due to the trauma, the child was now awake and upset during the overnight period (12 to 4 a.m.), her parents assumed that she was either hungry or needed extra comforting—so they started giving her a bottle.

In turn, the baby grew accustomed to that "new" bottle, and began to expect it every night. Soon enough, the previously clockwork-like sleeping schedule was a thing of the past.

Before they knew it, these parents were coming into our office for the *one-year* checkup and reporting that they still were giving the child this overnight bottle because it was the only thing that put her to sleep. You can't reintroduce an overnight feeding, for whatever reason, and then take it for granted that one day the child is going to wave that bottle away and say (or think), "I don't want it anymore."

One Final Note of Caution: Getting a child used to an overnight bottle even runs the risk of interfering with nighttime potty training down the line. The bladder can only hold so much liquid for so long; a child who is accustomed to drinking a lot overnight might end up having a more difficult time controlling her bladder when she's supposed to be in bed, asleep.

The Jassey Cocktail

In order to get your baby back on the right track after teething or another such trauma, in lieu of that "bottle Band-Aid," we recommend the "Jassey Cocktail."

While the occasional martini or glass of Pinot might be a welcome elixir to help smooth over the rough parts of baby rearing for some parents, that's not what we're talking about here.

The Jassey Cocktail is one or a combination of over-the-counter medicines that we have found extremely effective in treating teething babies, or babies who have experienced similar sleep-interfering traumas, and helping them get back on the right sleep track. (Make sure to check the dosage chart on page 107 for the minimum ages for each medicine, and always check with your pediatrician before giving your child any new medicines.)

The proper dosages vary, but the Cocktail is always one or a combination of the following:

- Acetaminophen (Tylenol)

- Ibuprofen (brand names include Advil and Motrin)

- Diphenhydramine (Benadryl)

IS BENADRYL "BABY AMBIEN"?

Some of the parents we work with don't bat an eye when we suggest Benadryl for its sleep-inducing properties; others ask questions like "Is Benadryl like baby Ambien?" The answer is no.

When given in appropriate doses, Benadryl is harmless. As proof of this, think about it the following way: If your baby suffered from an acute allergic reaction—one that was known to be alleviated by Benadryl—would you withhold that medicine from the child?

Similarly, if your child suffered from chronic allergies, there's a good chance you'd have to give her Benadryl every six hours. *That* would be considered healthy for the baby, so we daresay that one Benadryl dose per night for a few nights is unlikely to do any harm.

Benadryl is a perfectly legitimate way to temporarily help your baby reset the clock. In fact, it's something we can even be grateful for. After all, it was only one or two generations back when a dab of whiskey, administered on the gums, was deemed an acceptable method of putting an inconsolable infant to sleep.

The bottom line is that when adults fall into a rut of sleeplessness, they can usually correct it on their own by doing things like exercising, adjusting their diet, or reading baby sleep books.

But the infant child has no such alternatives. She needs something that is more certain to succeed.

Note on Homeopathic Alternatives: Some parents ask us about homeopathic alternatives to Benadryl, such as Hyland's Baby Teething Tablets. We caution them that for one thing, tablets don't easily dissolve, and the child might have difficulty getting them down. For another thing, homeopathic products are

MEDICATION DOSAGES

Acetaminophen (Tylenol) every 4 hours (Only for children at least 2 months old)	Children's Liquid Suspension/ New Infant Suspension (160 mg/5 ml) (½ tsp is 2.5 ml)
6–8 lbs	¼ tsp
9–11 lbs	⅓ tsp
12–17 lbs	½ tsp
18–22 lbs	¾ tsp
23–28 lbs	1 tsp
29–34 lbs	1¼ tsp
35–40 lbs	1½ tsp
Ibuprophen (Advil/Motrin) every 6 hours (Only for children at least 6 months old)	Children's Liquid Suspension (100 mg/5 ml)
12–16 lbs	½ tsp
17–21 lbs	¾ tsp
22–27 lbs	1 tsp
28–32 lbs	1¼ tsp
33–38 lbs	1½ tsp
Diphenhydramine (Benadryl) every 6 hours (Only for children at least 6 months old) NOTE: Benadryl can be mixed with ibuprophen, but not acetaminophen.	Children Suspension
10–15 lbs	½ tsp
16–21 lbs	¾ tsp
22–27 lbs	1 tsp
28–32 lbs	1¼ tsp
33–38 lbs	1½ tsp

not always subject to the same rigorous testing that's done on conventional medicines. Natural is not always better.

Note: 5 to 10 percent of children won't become drowsy from Benadryl; it will have the opposite effect on them. If you're lucky enough to have one of these children, you'll probably know it soon enough.

In the chart on page 107 are the dosages we recommend for the Jassey Cocktail, along with instructions on when to use it. *As always, consult your pediatrician before giving your child any medicines.*

WHEN TO SERVE IT

Give your baby the Jassey Cocktail right before bed. It may take a few nights to reset the clock; it may take around a week. (You can also use Orajel or Anbesol to help things along.) As long as you're using the proper dosages, all of these medicines are perfectly safe.

CHAPTER SEVEN

Let's Eat

Introducing Solid Foods

Solid Food Guidelines

As memorable as your baby's expressions are from day one, food will introduce still more amazing facial contortions of both pleasure and unease. Watching a human being try different foods for the first time is a priceless experience.

It is now commonly accepted by all major medical associations and other relevant organizations that most babies can begin to try solid foods between four and six months of age, or when they reach a body weight of fourteen pounds.* We recommend to the parents we see that they can start at four months, but there's certainly no harm in waiting a little while longer if you prefer. (We recommend not starting *before* four months be-

---

* An exception to this rule is mixing cereal with the milk to weigh it down to fight reflux.

cause newer studies have suggested an increased risk in future obesity in babies fed before that mark.)

As an alternative to starting at *precisely* four months, you can also wait until you notice your baby eyeing your own food; that's a good rule of thumb.

We have a couple of simple, general rules for introducing foods to your baby's diet:

1. *Introduce only one food every three days.* This is to make sure that if your baby has an allergic reaction to a particular food, we can be certain *which* food it is.

   For instance, if you introduce rice and oatmeal to your child at the same time, and she develops an allergic reaction some time later, it will be very difficult to tell which food was the problematic one. Waiting seventy-two hours to introduce each new food is a way of making sure there's no confusion on the allergy front.

2. *Similarly, we advise parents to introduce new foods in the morning/early afternoon.* If your child *does* experience a sudden allergic reaction or intolerance to a new food, it's safer to have the rest of the day to deal with it. Not to mention that this way, you're more likely to be awake if something happens.

Mix It Up, But One at a Time: We don't want to give the impression that you can only feed your baby one thing at a time if you're introducing a new food.

For instance, if you've successfully introduced bananas for three days, and then you want to bring pears into the mix, you don't have to feed your baby only pears for three days. You can feed her pears in the morning, and bananas in the afternoon, or even mix the two together. In fact, you can even introduce a new food as *part* of a mixture, if you like—so long as the food it's *being* mixed with has already been successfully incorporated into the child's diet.

Then be sure to wait seventy-two hours before introducing the *next* food.

Start Spooning

FIRST UP: CEREAL

Start with cereal. As you'll see in the following table, babies at least four months of age can also safely digest several fruits, as well as a few veggies, but cereal is doubtlessly the safest food to begin with: rice, oatmeal or even barley.

Begin by giving your child solid food twice a day, prior to a bottle or breast-feeding. As we said before, one of these feedings should be in the morning, so you can pin down any potential allergic reaction. Beyond that rule, you can choose whichever feedings are conducive to your schedule.

For each solid feeding, mix a tablespoon of dried cereal with *about* half an ounce of milk and feed your child with the spoon. Experiment with the texture using more or less milk; different babies go for different consistencies. This little meal should take your baby around five to ten minutes to "finish" (chances are that more than half of it will wind up *on* the child rather than *in* the child). Afterward, wash the mixture down with the regularly scheduled breast or bottle. The baby might not finish the bottle because she's full, which is perfectly fine.

NEXT LEVEL: FRUITS AND VEGGIES

After your child has been eating—and tolerating—cereal for at least a week, you can move on to fruits and/or vegetables. This is another area where different people—and doctors—have different preferences. As you'll see in the chart that follows, there are more than a few fruits a child should be able to digest at four months of age, and a few vegetables, but Lewis likes to introduce fruits at four months and wait until five months for the veggies. Jonathan is comfortable with bringing them into the fold at the same stage. It's up to you. Or more realistically, it's up to your child, as she will subtly—or not so subtly—guide you in the direction of certain foods.

The following table is a broad guide to which foods your child should be able to eat at certain stages of life.

Important Note: Foods that naturally contain some hard, rubbery or otherwise potentially choking element, like cucumbers, asparagus or zucchini, should always be *shredded, de-seeded* and *chopped finely* before serving. If you think it might need chewing—as opposed to *gumming*—don't give it to your baby as is.

Pureeing these foods is also a good, safe way to go.

4 MONTHS	5 MONTHS	6 MONTHS	9 MONTHS	1 YEAR
Cereals	**Fruits**	**Fruits**	**Fruits**	**Others**
Rice	Mango	Pomegranate	Cherries	Whole Milk
Oatmeal	Guava	Figs	Strawberries	Peanut Butter
Barley	Kiwi	**Meats**	Blueberries	Honey
Fruits	Papaya	Chicken	Raspberries	Non-Shellfish
Bananas	Avocado	Turkey	Pineapple	Shellfish
Applesauce	**Vegetables**	Beef	Oranges	
Pears	Corn	Lamb	Tomato	
Peaches	Peas	Veal	Grapefruit	
Apricots	Green Beans	Ham	**Vegetables**	
Plums	Spinach	**Others**	Beets	
Prunes	Zucchini	Mashed Potatoes	Peppers	
Grapes	Broccoli	Beans	Mushrooms	
Honeydew	Cauliflower	Cheeses	Olives	
Cantaloupe		Pastina/ Pastas	Cucumbers	
Watermelon		Teething Biscuits	Pickles	
Vegetables		Breads	**Others**	
Sweet Potatoes		Tapioca	Egg Yolk	
Carrots		Cheerios/ Puffs	Egg White	
Squash			Custards	
			Puddings	
			Jell-O	
			Chocolate	
			Ice Cream	
			Pancakes	
			French Toast	
			Waffles	
			Jelly	
			Pizza	

THE BLIZZARD RULE

We strongly advise parents to incorporate into their child's diet as many of these foundation foods as possible. And by *incorporate* we mean something a little more substantial than a brief broccoli drive-by or quick cauliflower cameo. We don't mean force-feeding your baby anything; let's call it *persistent prodding*. Again, remember you're a parent, not Burger King; your little one doesn't get to "have it her way." It's up to you to teach her what's good to eat.

We hear a lot of parents say something to the effect of "Well, I can't feed her vegetables, because she won't eat them, and she needs to eat *something*." Or maybe certain fruits are the issue, or beans, or rice. (You get the picture.)

We respond by explaining to these parents the Blizzard Rule:

If a blizzard hit your town, and you were stranded in your house for a few days, and couldn't go to the grocery store, and that vegetable or fruit in question was the only food you had to give your baby, what would you do?

You see what we're getting at? As we've said many times, taking care of a baby is such a visceral enterprise—where feelings and emotions often override logic, reason and science—that it's all too easy to lose sight of the greater good, the bigger picture, the more long-term goals. Sometimes it's a matter of changing your vantage point—of gaining some distance from the matter at hand, so you can deal with it in a rational manner.

THE FUTURE DINNER RULE

Along those lines, if you're not a fan of our blizzard rule, think of it this way:

Imagine your baby five, seven or ten years from now: a growing child. The whole family is sitting down to a delicious, home-cooked square meal: baked chicken, mashed potatoes, green beans and freshly baked rolls. The child is eating all of it—except for, you notice, the green beans. Come to think of it, this child never eats anything green. You implore her to pick up one string bean and to eat it. Just one (hoping it won't be too bad, and will lead to more). You beg. You plead. But she just won't budge.

"I just don't like vegetables," she says. "I can't eat them."

We're guessing you wouldn't tolerate that from a growing child, so why give up so easily with a baby—one who, one day, might *be* that green-averse kid?

It might take a surprisingly great number of feedings for your baby to activate certain taste buds and to discover the appeal of certain foods. She may recoil from spinach nineteen times in a row and then, miraculously, consume it willingly on the twentieth attempt.

We're not necessarily implying that you should give each and every food on that list twenty chances. You'll have to use your best judgment. But suffice it to say: You never know when a particular food might "take," and you owe it to your baby to give it the best chance possible.

After all, she's going to be judging foods by this palate for the rest of her life. It would be nice to give her a fighting chance.

Note: For the most part, children will like most any food you give them until around the age of two. But we like to invoke the Blizzard and Future Dinner rules for two reasons: (1) Babies might not take to a particular food at first because of some random reason, and we don't want you to misattribute it to that food, and (2) let's be real: Some of us *adults* don't like certain foods, and we hope you don't restrict your child's diet on account of the limitations of your own.

Portions

As you may already know, or as you'll soon find out, commercial baby foods are divided into "stages"; some brands use that word specifically, and others use slightly different terminology, referring to certain foods as "beginner" foods or "1st" foods. "Since these stages aren't standardized, the American Academy of Pediatrics, in their *Guide to Your Child's Nutrition*, advises that "two rules apply across the board: Begin with stage 1 foods for beginners, and don't offer your child toddler foods, which often contain chunks, until he is an experienced eater."[1]

The various brands of baby food define their stages differently, but as a general rule, here's what to expect from each stage:

STAGE 1: Single-ingredient foods; pureed fruits and vegetables

STAGE 2: Single-ingredient foods; combination foods

STAGE 3: More textured foods, with more complex flavors; foods with small chunks

STAGE 4: This usually refers to "table food," meaning the food the rest of the family eats—whether or not the child is actually at the table.

Different children will progress through these stages at different rates. Use your best judgment and let your child progress to each successive stage after she's proven herself "comfortable" with the foods in the previous one.

As a *general* rule, "Stage 1" containers are usually somewhere around two ounces, "Stage 2" containers are around four ounces, and "Stage 3" containers are around six ounces.

Make sure your child's gums are sufficiently hard before moving to Stage 3 foods, which are more textured and may contain larger chunks than she's used to.

Age	Stage	Portion Size / Frequency
4–5 months	Stage 1	½–full container (2–3 tbsp) / 1–2 times per day
6–9 months	Stage 2	½–full container (¼–½ cup) / 2–3 times per day
9–12 months	Stage 3	½–full container (½ cup) / 3 times per day
1 year +	Almost exclusively table food	Note: Table food can be introduced sooner than one year. If it's really soft, table food can be introduced as early as six months.

Switching from Breast Milk or Formula to Whole Milk

Around twelve months of age, you should also introduce your baby to whole milk for proper brain development.

For some children, this switch will be seamless. Literally just a matter of substituting whole milk for formula.

If your baby "rejects" the whole milk, try a slower transition. Fill the bottle—or sippy cup—with ¼ whole milk and ¾ formula. The next week, move on to half formula, half milk. Then the third week, use a ¾ milk, ¼ formula ratio. Finally, in week four, eliminate formula altogether.

Since eating and sleeping are so closely linked, it's important to help your child's diet develop in a deliberate, wholesome way, so you don't undo any of the healthy sleeping habits she's learned so far.

In the next chapter, we discuss the need to get your baby to switch from the bottle to the sippy cup at around one year as well. We recommend that you avoid switching to whole milk and from bottle to sippy cup at the same time. If the child has an adverse reaction, you won't know which new element caused it. (Additionally, it's always best to make one big change at a time, so it's more easily assimilated.) Decide which switch you want to make first, then space these two transitions a week or two apart.

CHAPTER EIGHT

Common Questions, Sample Schedules and Well Baby Exams

FAQs

SHOULD I BE CONCERNED ABOUT SIDS?

Since 1994, when the National Institute of Child Health and Human Development launched the "Back to Sleep" campaign—which recommends that babies sleep on their backs or sides, rather than stomachs—the rate of sudden infant death syndrome (SIDS) in the United States has plunged 50 percent.[1]

SIDS is fortunately *extremely rare*, occurring at a rate of fewer than one death for every one thousand births, or less than 0.1 percent.

Pacifiers and ceiling fans have also proven effective in fighting SIDS. The prevailing theory is that some babies don't have fully developed startle reflexes, and that when they are in deep sleep, they are therefore extra-susceptible to overheating or suffocating from pillows or other objects. Pacifiers and ceiling fans might serve to prevent these children from falling into too-deep sleep, thusly helping to protect them from SIDS.

Keep your baby off her stomach and don't give SIDS a second thought.

By the Way: When your baby can roll over in both directions, she *can* be put on her stomach. You might still want to avoid placing her in the crib that way, just to be safe, but hopefully that knowledge will give you a wider perspective on the issue.

HOW OFTEN SHOULD MY BABY POOP?

As we mentioned earlier, in Chapter 3, a baby could move her bowels once a week and, if she shows no signs of distress, be perfectly healthy. On the other hand, an infant might produce perfect pellets three times a day like a machine and suffer from gastrointestinal issues just the same. Along with everything else with babies, we need to view bowel movements from a big-picture perspective. You have to take into consideration the baby's mood, eating habits and other factors.

Here are two rules of thumb we can share with confidence:

- The more babies poop, the better they tend to feel, since they are more frequently getting rid of gas.

- If your baby seems to be pooping in an abnormal manner for five consecutive days, you should contact a doctor. What's abnormal? Use your best, big-picture judgment.

HOW HIGH A FEVER IS TOO HIGH?

If your baby runs a fever of at least 100.4 degrees before four to eight weeks of age, the commonly accepted standard in pediatrics calls for her to be admitted to the hospital for a comprehensive battery of tests. This is required as a precaution because at that extremely young age, infants have underdeveloped immune systems* and are susceptible to certain life-threatening illnesses, including bacteremia, urinary tract infections, and meningitis. To protect against those diseases, the hospital will run a triad of tests on the infant: They'll do blood work, insert a urinary catheter and perform a spinal tap.

If your baby is two months or older and running a fever, try to consider it from a big-picture perspective. We are more concerned by an infant whose temperature is 101 degrees but who looks, to put it bluntly, terrible, than we are by a baby with a higher fever who does not appear to be in distress.

So if your baby is running a fever and is listless and lethargic, contact your doctor immediately. But if she has only a slight fever and otherwise seems fine, chances are that she is.

In general, fevers pose a risk to babies when they rise or fall rapidly; large fluctuations are more of a threat to a baby's health than a high temperature by itself. Please bear that in mind, as well. (That precipitous rise and fall is what causes febrile seizures, incidentally.)

---

* Over the first six months of life, infants live off their mother's antibodies, which they acquired while in the womb. These inherited antibodies dissipate as the baby's body starts manufacturing its own; this turnover compromises the immune system.

In addition to calling your physician if your baby runs a fever, or is inconsolable for a lengthy period of time, you may place her in a lukewarm bath to help bring her temperature down. But that is the extent of what you can do without the aid of a doctor.

Note on Fever Reducers: If the child is over two months, you can give her acetaminophen (Tylenol).

You must wait until six months of age to administer ibuprofen (Advil, Motrin); before then, the child's kidneys are not developed enough to process it.

IS THIS RASH OK?

Rashes are the most difficult baby ailment to diagnose over the phone or, as it were, in the pages of a book. To make matters more complicated, red spots and blotches are super-common on healthy babies; it can be easy to misread an ordinary—and temporary—skin inconsistency as a rash.

If an unusual mark or blotch is accompanied by a high fever, is not improving or is otherwise concerning to you, contact your pediatrician. If you suspect the irregularity may be a typical result of babyhood, it probably is!

Sample Daily Schedules

Some parents might find it helpful to know the broad parameters outlining how much their child should be eating, *what* she should be eating, and how much she should be sleeping every day. Here are some general guidelines for each three-month stage of life, from just-born to fifteen months. Remember that no two babies are alike, so yours may well deviate from these "norms" and still be perfectly healthy. These are references, not rules.

0–3 MONTHS

Feed only breast milk or formula. The total amount per day is variable, depending on weight and the frequency of feedings.

Breast

Nurse eight to twelve times a day (every two to three hours) *until milk supply has come in*. After that, work your way up to feeding every four hours by increasing the time between feedings by fifteen minutes per day.

Efficient breast-feeders will spend fifteen to twenty minutes per breast.

Formula

Feed every four hours or work up to four hours by increasing the time between feedings fifteen minutes per day.

Multiply baby weight by 2.25 for a rough estimate of the total number of ounces per day. Infants can take anywhere from two to eight ounces per feed depending on age.

The overall goals for both groups is to feed five times a day and to go around eight hours from the final feeding of the night to the first feeding the next morning.

Once the child is consistently sleeping around eight hours per night, you can try to extend that to twelve hours by eliminating the final night feeding, so that you're feeding four times per day. Do this by pushing the final night feeding forward fifteen minutes and the first morning feeding back by fifteen minutes, per day, until that final night feeding gets close enough to the one before it to become unnecessary.

4-6 MONTHS

Start to introduce solid foods twice a day: cereals, then fruits and veggies. Wash them down with a bottle or breast milk. (The child might take a little less milk during those feedings.)

Introduce foods one at a time, waiting seventy-two hours between foods to monitor any allergic reactions. And always start a new food in the morning so someone is awake to look for possible reactions, and so you have the rest of the day to respond.

Breast-fed children might become more efficient and nurse more quickly (five to fifteen minutes per breast).

Formula-fed children will take anywhere from four to eight ounces per feed.

The goal is to go twelve hours between feedings overnight, and eight hours at least. Four or five feedings total per day.

7-9 MONTHS

Feed the child three solid meals per day, possibly dropping one bottle/breast-feeding. The baby can have two snacks per day as well.

Introduce the sippy cup, so she can start getting used to it.

Start meats and some easy textured foods.

Breast-fed babies may now feed as little as five minutes per breast.

Formula-fed babies will take around fifteen to twenty ounces total per day.

10–12 MONTHS

Keep feeding your baby *only* breast milk or formula (the kidneys aren't ready to process whole milk yet).

Breast-fed babies will continue to feed quickly—around five minutes per breast.

Formula-fed babies will take around fifteen to twenty ounces total per day.

Three meals and two snacks per day.

Encourage her to eat more textured foods and less baby food, which will help incite her to develop her pincer grasp—using the fingers and thumb to pick up an object—because she'll want to pick up foods like cheerios or crackers.

Start using the sippy cup even more. Try to get the child completely off the bottle by the one-year mark.

13–15 MONTHS

Switch to whole milk, which aids brain development—but no more than sixteen to twenty-four ounces per day. If your child doesn't like milk, then you can give her anything with dairy at least two to three times per day.

Ditch the bottle and pacifier.

Ditch baby foods and feed only table foods.

One Year: Bye-Bye Bottle (and Binky)

We recommend that parents wean their babies off of the bottle and pacifier by the one-year mark. There are three main reasons for this:

- *Behavior:* The longer you wait, the harder it will be for the child to break the habit. And at around fifteen to eighteen months of age, a child is vulnerable to becoming strongly attached to a bottle or pacifier, so we'd prefer to liberate her from them long before then.

- *Ear infections:* The Eustachian tubes, which link the ears to the upper respiratory system, are basically horizontal in kids, whereas they are at inclines in adults. So if a child is congested, that fluid can leak through the tubes to the ears and cause an infection. Sucking can facilitate this, particularly if the child is lying down with the bottle.

- *Bottle rot (tooth decay):* Tooth decay can occur when the baby teeth are exposed to prolonged contact with sugars found in milk, formula, juice or soda. The bottle has the potential to facilitate this prolonged exposure (for instance, the child might fall asleep with the bottle in her mouth).

ELIMINATING THE BEDTIME BOTTLE

Sometimes when we tell parents they should ditch the bottle by the twelve-month mark, they say they can't, because the before-bed bottle is the only way they can get their child to sleep. They can eliminate every other bottle, but not that last one.

We sympathize. In this kind of scenario, we recommend patience and persistence more than anything. A child who resists the sippy cup one, two, three or even several nights in a row might take it after a week or so. This may disrupt the bedtime routine a bit, but it's worth it.

In addition to patience and persistence, you might also try tweaking the bedtime routine a little. For instance, if you usually read your little one a story or sing to her, then give her the bottle, then put her in bed, try giving her the sippy cup *during* the story or singing. Give her a little more time with it. Or, if reading or singing or something similar is *not* part of the routine, try adding it along with the sippy cup. A little misdirection.

Just bear in mind that it's important to keep *most* of the bedtime routine the same as it's always been; as we've said, too much change at once can be difficult for babies. They thrive on routine, hence our primary recommendation of patience. But do know that along with patience, a small tweak can go a long way.

Also please remember that getting rid of the bottle is just another unavoidable test of adaptation. All children have to adapt to a multitude of adjustments, including getting off the bottle, getting off the pacifier, getting out of diapers and graduating from the crib. These challenges are inevitable—know that the longer you wait to address them, the more difficult they will be.

"WHAT DO I DO IF MY CHILD IS NOW NOT TAKING ANY MILK WHATSOEVER?"

Occasionally, parents will tell us that without the bottle, their child won't drink any milk at all—even out of a sippy cup.

We totally sympathize.

We tell these parents that, believe it or not, getting zero milk per day can be absolutely fine for a one-year-old—*as long as she's getting two to three servings of a suitable replacement.*

Indeed, a growing child needs calcium, but sufficient quantities of that mineral are found in plenty of other sources, including yogurts, cheeses, animal crackers, cereal bars, yogurt milk, bread, Ovaltine and countless additional foods.

Believe it or not, even some brands of orange juice have more calcium than milk.

Well Baby Exams

The APA's guidelines recommend examinations for newborns at two weeks, one month, two months, four months, six months, nine months, one year, fifteen months, eighteen months, and two years.

In our practice, we like to see new parents and their babies when the child is a week or so old, and then at one month and every month thereafter until six months; after that, we like to see them at nine months and one year.

We understand that some health insurance plans might not allow for that many visits; we simply mention it as an ideal.

At any rate, it might be helpful for you to see what we look for in these newborn examinations. What follows are reproductions of the checklists we go over at these visits.

After all, don't you wish you could always get a look at the examination ahead of time?

NEWBORN

Parent/Guardian Questionnaire

■ PREGNANCY, LABOR AND DELIVERY

Were there any problems during your pregnancy?

....

....

How long was your labor? ....

What type of delivery did you have—vaginal or C-section?

....

Were there any problems during the delivery?

....

Did your baby go into the NICU? ....

Did the infant receive the hepatitis B vaccine at birth?

....

■ FEEDING

My baby is breast-feeding/bottle feeding/formula feeding.

....

My baby breast-feeds for .... minutes on each side every ....
hours.

My baby takes .... ounces of .... formula every .... hours.

Is your child fussy or irritable after feeding? ....

Does your child spit up a lot after feeding? ....

How many diapers per day for urine ....   stools ....

■ SLEEPING

My baby sleeps back/side. ....

Where does your baby sleep? ....

■ DEVELOPMENT

You may have noticed that your baby:

☐ Looks at your face
☐ Lifts head up
☐ Hears your voice
☐ Grasps your finger

Have you noticed any yellow color to your baby's skin?

....

■ EDUCATION/ANTICIPATORY GUIDANCE

- ☐ Car seat (rear facing)
- ☐ Feeding patterns
- ☐ Family adjustment
- ☐ Bathing
- ☐ Umbilical cord care
- ☐ Sleeping (You should ace this one at the very least!)
- ☐ Circumcision care (if applicable)
- ☐ Fever
- ☐ Crib safety

Follow up at one month unless otherwise noted.

1 MONTH

Parent/Guardian Questionnaire

Do you have any questions or concerns?..

■ DIET

My baby is breast-feeding/bottle feeding/formula feeding.

....

My baby breast-feeds for .... minutes on each side every ....
hours.

My baby takes .... ounces of .... formula every .... hours.

Is your child fussy or irritable after feeding? ....

Does your child spit up a lot after feeding? ....

How many diapers per day for urine ....   stools ....

Does your baby get constipated? ....

■ DEVELOPMENT

You may have noticed that your baby:

☐   Turns to your voice
☐   Lifts head while on tummy
☐   Coos
☐   Smiles

■ SLEEP

Where does your baby sleep? ....

How many hours straight does your baby sleep at night?

....

How many hours in total does your baby sleep at night?

....

■ **EDUCATION/ANTICIPATORY GUIDANCE**

☐ Fever/illnesses

☐ Immunization reactions

☐ Car seat (rear facing)

☐ Feeding patterns

☐ Sleep position

☐ Tummy time

☐ Rolling over

☐ Crib safety

☐ Circumcision care (if applicable)

Follow up at two months unless otherwise noted.

2 MONTHS

Parent/Guardian Questionnaire

Do you have any questions or concerns?..

■ **DIET**

My baby is breast-feeding/bottle feeding/formula feeding.
....

My baby breast-feeds for .... minutes on each side every ....
hours.

My baby takes .... ounces of .... formula every .... hours.

Is your child fussy or irritable after feeding? ....

Does your child spit up a lot after feeding? ....

How many diapers per day for urine .... stools ....

Does your baby get constipated? ....

■ **DEVELOPMENT**

You may have noticed that your baby:

☐ Smiles
☐ Lifts head while on tummy
☐ Follows objects to the middle
☐ Brings hand to mouth
☐ Coos

■ **SLEEP**

Where does your baby sleep? ....

Does your baby sleep on her back or on her side?

....

How many hours straight does your baby sleep at night? ....

How many hours in total does your baby sleep at night?

....

■ **EDUCATION/ANTICIPATORY GUIDANCE**

☐ Fever/illnesses

☐ Immunization reactions

☐ Car seat (rear facing)

☐ Feeding patterns

☐ Sleep position

☐ Tummy time

☐ Rolling over

Follow up at three months unless otherwise noted.

3 MONTHS

Parent/Guardian Questionnaire

Do you have any questions or concerns?..

■ **DIET**

My baby is breast-feeding/bottle feeding/formula feeding.

....

My baby breast-feeds for .... minutes on each side every .... hours.

My baby takes .... ounces of .... formula every .... hours.

Is your child fussy or irritable after feeding? ....

Does your child spit up a lot after feeding? ....

How many diapers per day for urine .... stools ....

Does your baby get constipated? ....

■ **DEVELOPMENT**

You may have noticed your baby:

☐ Starting to focus across the room when on tummy

☐ Smiles

☐ Follows objects past the middle

☐ Coos

☐ Reaches for and/or grasps objects

☐ Lifts head while on tummy

☐ Brings hand to mouth

■ **SLEEP**

Does your baby sleep on her back or on her side?

....

How many hours straight does your baby sleep at night? ....

How many hours in total does your baby sleep at night?

....

■ EDUCATION/ANTICIPATORY GUIDANCE

☐ Fever/illnesses

☐ Immunization reactions

☐ Car seat (rear facing)

☐ No bottle propping

☐ Sleep position

☐ Tummy time

☐ Rolling over

☐ Playpen safety

☐ Introducing cereals

Follow up at four months unless otherwise noted.

4 MONTHS

Parent/Guardian Questionnaire

Do you have any questions or concerns?...

■ DIET

My baby is breast-feeding/bottle feeding/formula feeding.

....

My baby breast-feeds for .... minutes on each side every ....
hours.

My baby takes .... ounces of .... formula every .... hours.

Has your baby started eating cereals? ....

Does your baby get constipated? ....

■ DEVELOPMENT

You may have noticed your baby:

- ☐ Transfers objects from one hand to the other
- ☐ Rolls over
- ☐ Plays with a rattle
- ☐ Looks for dropped objects
- ☐ Has elbows out and head up while on tummy
- ☐ Laughs, gurgles, squeals

■ SLEEP

How many hours does your child sleep at night?

....

Is your baby sleeping through the night? ....

■ EDUCATION/ANTICIPATORY GUIDANCE

- ☐ Fever/illnesses
- ☐ Introducing cereals
- ☐ Car seat (rear facing)
- ☐ Introducing fruits/juices
- ☐ Sleep position
- ☐ Teething

- ☐ Rolling over
- ☐ Playpen safety
- ☐ Immunization reactions

Follow up at five months unless otherwise noted.

5 MONTHS

Parent/Guardian Questionnaire

Do you have any questions or concerns?......................................

■ DIET

My baby is breast-feeding/bottle feeding/formula feeding.

....

My baby breast-feeds for .... minutes on each side every ....
hours.

My baby takes .... ounces of .... formula every .... hours.

Has your baby started eating cereals? ....

Has your child had any reactions to foods? ....

Does your baby get constipated? ....

■ DEVELOPMENT

You may have noticed your baby:

- ☐ Transfers objects from one hand to the other
- ☐ Rolls over
- ☐ Plays with a rattle
- ☐ Looks for dropped objects
- ☐ Has elbows out and head up while on tummy
- ☐ Bears weight

■ SLEEP

How many hours does your child sleep at night? ....

Is your baby sleeping through the night? ....

■ EDUCATION/ANTICIPATORY GUIDANCE

- ☐ Fever/illnesses
- ☐ Introducing cereals
- ☐ Car seat (rear facing)
- ☐ Introducing fruits/juices
- ☐ Sleep position
- ☐ Teething
- ☐ Rolling over
- ☐ Playpen safety
- ☐ Immunization reactions

Follow up at six months unless otherwise noted.

6 MONTHS

Parent/Guardian Questionnaire

Do you have any questions or concerns?..

■ **DIET**

My baby is breast-feeding/bottle feeding/formula feeding.
....

My baby breast-feeds for .... minutes on each side every ....
hours.

My baby takes .... ounces of .... formula every .... hours.

List some fruits and vegetables your child has eaten.
....

Has your child had any reactions to foods? ....

Does your child get constipated? ....

■ **DEVELOPMENT**

You may have noticed that your child:

☐ Takes and holds two objects
☐ Bears weight

- [ ] Passes objects from hand to hand
- [ ] Rakes small objects
- [ ] "Raspberries"
- [ ] Sits with support
- [ ] Rolls over
- [ ] Babbles and laughs
- [ ] Sits without support
- [ ] Has arms outstretched and head up when on belly

▪ SLEEP

Do you have trouble getting your child to sleep?

....

▪ EDUCATION/ANTICIPATORY GUIDANCE

- [ ] Fever/illnesses
- [ ] Immunization reactions
- [ ] Car seat (rear facing)
- [ ] Bedtime routine
- [ ] Sippy cup
- [ ] Introducing proteins
- [ ] Childproofing
- [ ] Introducing vegetables
- [ ] Separation anxiety
- [ ] Advice against walkers

Follow up at nine months unless otherwise noted.

9 MONTHS

Parent/Guardian Questionnaire

Do you have any questions or concerns?...

■ **DIET**

My baby is breast-feeding/bottle feeding/formula feeding.

....

My baby breast-feeds for .... minutes on each side every ....
hours.

My baby takes .... ounces of .... formula every .... hours.

List some foods your child likes to eat. ....

Has your child had any reactions to foods? ....

Does your child get constipated?...

■ **DEVELOPMENT**

You may have noticed that your child:

- ☐ Crawls
- ☐ Pulls to a standing position
- ☐ Stands holding on
- ☐ Cruises along furniture

- ☐ Reaches for toys
- ☐ Bangs things together
- ☐ Uses a pincer grasp
- ☐ Babbles and laughs
- ☐ Indicates wants by vocalizing
- ☐ Waves bye-bye
- ☐ Finger feeds
- ☐ Gives high-fives/patty-cake motion
- ☐ Makes good eye contact
- ☐ Imitates speech, jabbers: "mama," "dada," "baba"

■ **SLEEP**

Where does your baby sleep? ....

Does your baby sleep on her back or side? ....

Is your baby sleeping through the night? ....

■ **EDUCATION/ANTICIPATORY GUIDANCE**

- ☐ Fever/illnesses
- ☐ Immunization reactions
- ☐ Car seat (rear facing)
- ☐ Feeding patterns
- ☐ Sleep position
- ☐ Tummy time
- ☐ Rolling over

Follow up at one year unless otherwise noted.

1 YEAR

Parent/Guardian Questionnaire

Do you have any questions or concerns?..

■ **DIET**

How much does your child drink? ....

How much juice does your child drink? ....

Is your child using a sippy cup? ....

List some foods your child likes to eat. ....

Has your child had any reactions to foods? ....

Does your child get constipated? ....

■ **DEVELOPMENT**

You may have noticed that your child:

☐ Pulls to a standing position
☐ Cruises along furniture
☐ Stands holding on
☐ Clasps hands
☐ Walks with hands held

- ☐ Walks alone
- ☐ Uses a neat pincer grasp
- ☐ Can speak a few words
- ☐ Says "mama" and "dada"
- ☐ Follows simple commands
- ☐ Indicates wants by pointing
- ☐ Responds to name
- ☐ Waves bye-bye
- ☐ Makes good eye contact
- ☐ Gives high-fives/patty-cake motion
- ☐ Shows affection

List some words your child says. ....

■ SLEEP

Where does your baby sleep? ....

Does your baby sleep on her back or side? ....

Is your baby sleeping through the night? ....

■ EDUCATION/ANTICIPATORY GUIDANCE

- ☐ Fever/illnesses
- ☐ Teething/dental health
- ☐ Car seat (forward facing)
- ☐ Food safety
- ☐ Immunization reactions

- ☐ Weaning from bottle
- ☐ Childproofing
- ☐ Normal decreased appetite

Follow up at fifteen months unless otherwise noted.

15 MONTHS

Parent/Guardian Questionnaire

Do you have any questions or concerns?...

■ **DIET**

How much milk does your child drink? ....

How much juice does your child drink? ....

Is your child drinking from a bottle? When? ....

Is your child using a sippy cup? ....

List some foods your child likes to eat. ....

Has your child had any reactions to foods? ....

Does your child get constipated? ....

■ DEVELOPMENT

You may have noticed that your child:

- ☐ Crawls up stairs
- ☐ Imitates housework
- ☐ Tries to feed self with spoon
- ☐ Speaks three to five words
- ☐ Walks with hands held
- ☐ Walks alone
- ☐ Plays alongside other kids
- ☐ Responds to name
- ☐ Scribbles
- ☐ Makes good eye contact
- ☐ Waves bye-bye
- ☐ Shows affection
- ☐ Gives high-fives/patty-cake motion

List some words your child says. ....

■ EDUCATION/ANTICIPATORY GUIDANCE

- ☐ Fever/illnesses
- ☐ Teething/dental health
- ☐ Car seat (forward facing)
- ☐ Food safety
- ☐ Immunization reactions
- ☐ Bedtime routine
- ☐ Childproofing
- ☐ Weaning from bottle

Follow up at eighteen months unless otherwise noted.

18 MONTHS

Parent/Guardian Questionnaire

Do you have any questions or concerns?..

■ **DIET**

How much milk does your child drink? ....

How much juice does your child drink? ....

Is your child drinking from a bottle? When? ....

Is your child using a sippy cup? ....

List some foods your child likes to eat. ....

Has your child had any reactions to foods? ....

Does your child get constipated? ....

■ **DEVELOPMENT**

You may have noticed that your child:

☐   Is aware of bowel movements
☐   Scribbles
☐   Feeds self with spoon/fork
☐   Speaks four to ten words

☐ Follows two- to three-step commands

☐ Takes off shoes

☐ Plays alongside other kids

☐ Walks alone

☐ Holds glass without spilling

☐ Throws a ball overhand

☐ Waves bye-bye

☐ Shows affection

☐ Kicks a ball

☐ Combines words

List some words your child says. ....

■ **EDUCATION/ANTICIPATORY GUIDANCE**

☐ Fever/illnesses

☐ Teething/dental health

☐ Car seat (forward facing)

☐ Potty training

☐ Bedtime routine

☐ Childproofing

☐ Immunization reactions

Follow up at two years unless otherwise noted.

2 YEARS

Parent/Guardian Questionnaire

Do you have any questions or concerns?...

■ **DIET**

How much milk does your child drink? ....

How much juice does your child drink? ....

List some foods your child likes to eat. ....

Has your child had any reactions to foods? ....

Does your child get constipated? ....

■ **DEVELOPMENT**

You may have noticed that your child:

☐ Is aware of bowel movements
☐ Feeds self
☐ Goes up and down stairs
☐ Opens doors
☐ Helps with getting undressed
☐ Draws
☐ Combines two or more words
☐ Names one color
☐ Interacts well with other kids
☐ Throws a ball overhand
☐ Kicks a ball
☐ Jumps

List some words your child says. ....

Have you started potty training? ....

◾ EDUCATION/ANTICIPATORY GUIDANCE

- ☐ Fever/illnesses
- ☐ Teething/dental health
- ☐ Car seat (forward facing)
- ☐ Potty training
- ☐ Bedtime routine
- ☐ Childproofing
- ☐ Nutrition and dietary habits
- ☐ Physical activity/exercise

Follow up at three years unless otherwise noted.

CHAPTER NINE

Parent Testimonials

Sometimes the most effective instruction is the example of someone who's gone before you.

We asked some of the parents we see in our practice, who sleep trained their children with the Jassey Way, to share their experiences for this book.

The following stories are told in their own words and lightly edited for context and flow.

The New Parents Who Didn't Know What to Expect

LIZ AND BRYAN L.

When we met Dr. Lewis Jassey, we were about to be first-time parents and we were freaked out about everything. We weren't sure about how to do anything.

We met Lewis at our son Brady's first checkup, around a week after he was born. Everything looked fine. He was the perfect weight and everything else.

Then Lewis asked us how we were doing with feeding him.

I was breast-feeding Brady and so far, it had been going well I told him.

"How frequently are you feeding him?" Lewis asked.

I didn't know how frequently exactly, but I knew it wasn't every four hours, as Lewis would recommend.

"This is our first baby," I said. "We didn't think to put the feedings on any sort of schedule. It's probably around every two hours."

We were playing it by ear and going with the flow, trying to figure out what worked and what didn't. We weren't feeding "on demand," but it was pretty close to that.

"I am going to give you some advice, and I just want you to *try* it," Lewis said. "You may have heard about people rearranging their lives to adjust to their babies. But I don't believe that's how it should be. Your baby is new to your lives, and you're new to his life, but so is everything else right now for him. Meanwhile, you've been living your lives a certain way for years and years. It's the baby who should adjust to *your* life."

My husband, Bryan, and I looked at Lewis like he was crazy. Not a little crazy. Completely out of his mind. Like, *Do we need to start looking for a new doctor?* out of his mind.

"I think you should make it your goal to feed the baby every four hours," Lewis said. "Make that your goal, and work up to it. If you can get Brady to adjust to that schedule, your lives will be so much easier. Everything will be so much easier."

Then my husband, Bryan, spoke up, saying what we both were thinking.

"Wait a minute," he said. "Everything we've heard is that you're supposed to stop everything and do whatever your baby tells you."

That's all I had heard up to that point; that when you have a baby, it's like *your* life is essentially over. Lewis was coming at it from a completely different point of view. The things he was saying were never what I would have expected to hear from a pediatrician.

"Remember, your baby is a little human," Lewis said. "And humans adapt."

Lewis laid out a goal of Brady going four hours between feedings, and he told us to start out by just extending our current time between feedings by ten to fifteen minutes each day. He wanted us to go step-by-step, not making any big changes on any particular day.

It was like an epiphany for Bryan and me. We had only had Brady for a week at that point, but we were already beginning to feel a little worn down. We didn't know what to expect going forward, and here was this doctor saying it was all going to be okay; our baby was going to be fine, and we were going to be fine.

"But you need to figure it out for the baby," Lewis said. "Not the other way around."

We started following Lewis's advice as soon as we got home that day. I don't know how long it took, but it wasn't very long. Within a month or two, Brady was eating every four hours, and we didn't feel unsure of when we were supposed to feed him. We weren't playing it by ear anymore; we felt totally in control of the situation.

And the nighttime was going great, too. At first, our last feeding was at 11:30 or 12 at night. But sometime after we started sleep training—I don't remember how or when it happened, exactly—that last feeding became 8 p.m. Brady would go to sleep after that, and we wouldn't wake up during the night at all.

After that, having the baby in our lives didn't feel as difficult as we had expected. Of course, there were moments when it was tough. But the routine Lewis taught us gave us so much stability. We almost never felt overwhelmed.

Lewis was absolutely right. Brady fit right into the way we were already living; we didn't have to change the way we were living to fit Brady. For instance, we could occasionally go out at night, and we were able to take him; we didn't have to worry about some crazy outburst. We felt like we were always prepared.

We noticed a difference between our experience with Brady and the experience of parents we knew who were literally feeding their children on demand until they were one year old.

Several years later, when we had our second child—our daughter Katie—we started with the four-hour feeding rule from the get-go. It took a little while longer to get it right with Katie, but no longer than two months or so.

And we fed our children every which way: breast-feeding, pumping breast milk and bottle feeding, and formula feeding. But no matter how we were feeding, we knew we were "covered" if we stuck to the four-hour rule. It removed the uncertainty as to whether we were feeding *enough*.

Bryan and I made a good team. We've become huge advocates of not feeding a baby during the night, and feeding every four hours during the day. We tell any new parents we know that that schedule is the best parenting advice we ever got. We tell them we started a week after our first baby was born, and we've never looked back. We try to convert them all.

We had a neighbor who was proud that her third child was feeding every three hours. We suggested that she try to stretch it out every day by fifteen minutes, until she got to every four hours.

Bryan later bumped into her and she grabbed his arm and pulled him in close and said, "Bryan, I just have to thank you for your advice. Now we're feeding every four hours, and it's the greatest thing ever. We know exactly when he's going to eat, and we can plan around it."

It was exactly the same epiphany we had had. The realization that having a newborn doesn't have to lead to some out-of-control way of living. That you can still have your freedom. Not all the freedom you had *before* having a baby, but a lot more than you would have thought possible.

The Jassey Way was nothing short of life-changing for us.

Bryan likes to joke that it's a shame that the Jassey Way is only for babies.

"I wish," he says, "that they'd come up with a system for teenagers."

The Mom Who Absolutely Had to Get Her Whole Family on Board

CHRISTINA A.

When my son Nicholas was born three years ago, I needed to find a good pediatrician. I'm a nurse, and one of my colleagues at the hospital recommended Jonathan Jassey. Jonathan taught me his sleep training method, and I started it immediately. It didn't take that long to get Nicholas sleeping through the night. It was six weeks at the most. It felt easy.

But my four-month-old, Michael, was a different story. When he was born, we immediately started trying to regulate his sleeping cycle, and to go every four hours for feedings during the day.

But every two hours that Michael would go without a bottle, he'd start screaming, almost inconsolably. The only thing that would calm him down at all would be the bottle. And you could forget about him sleeping through the night. That wasn't happening either. As long as I had given Nicholas an extra ounce of milk for his last feeding, he'd sleep through the night. But not this child. I'd try to give Michael an extra ounce, but he wouldn't take any extra milk, period. And he'd always wake up during the night. I tried everything to get him to go back to sleep, but nothing would ever work. Finally I would just give him another bottle. That was the only thing that ever seemed to soothe him.

Finally, I was able to stretch it out to four hours during the daytime.

Then just before my maternity leave was up and I had to go back to work, Michael started sleeping eight hours during the night. This was after about three months.

As a nurse, I had a special reason for wanting Michael to be able to sleep through the night: my erratic schedule. Going back to work meant I'd be spending a lot of days and nights at the hospital; during most of those times, my parents would be looking after my sons, not me. My work schedule didn't give me much wiggle room. I would never have time to adjust to Michael's schedule; he had to adjust to mine. My parents *had* to be on the same page as me. While Michael was staying with them, my parents couldn't go "backward" on his sleep training.

But that last part was tough. When Michael was with me, if he woke up in the middle of the night, or if he cried at all between feedings, I always had the strength to wait him out without giving him milk. I would just give him the binky or put him in the stroller and roll him around or find another way of soothing him. But I would never feed him. It was just a matter of finding *anything else* to soothe him. I understood what I was working toward; I had my experience with Nicholas to remind me that having a baby that can sleep through the night makes your life so much easier. And I knew how disastrous it could be if I went back to work and Michael's sleep habits were getting worse, not better.

But my parents were a different story. In their minds, if a baby was crying, and feeding him would soothe him, then that's what you did. They didn't necessarily see the importance of working toward a larger goal.

So I had to frequently re-explain, and remind them of, what we were working toward.

"What's the big deal if we give him the bottle a little early?" my parents would ask. "It's only twenty minutes or so. It doesn't seem like it could make a real difference."

"Twenty minutes is not much to us," I'd (try to) calmly explain. "But in a baby's brain, that's a long time. If Michael knows that he can get milk by crying twenty minutes earlier, then he's never going to get on a schedule. He's going to want milk whenever he feels like it, instead of when he needs it. You're going to turn us all into a twenty-four-hour drive-thru!"

That was one thing that Jonathan always impressed upon me; that I didn't have to be "open" all the time for my baby. It was just a matter of retraining his brain to know what his stomach knew; if he already had the right amount of calories for the day, he'd be absolutely fine without food until the morning. If I—or my parents—gave him a couple of ounces of milk during the nighttime, he might go back to bed, but it wouldn't achieve anything in the long run. His sleep habits might get worse, all so he could get milk he didn't need in the first place. And it was the same during the day; Michael could only be an efficient sleeper at night if he was an efficient eater during the day; it was so important for him to feed every four hours.

I had come to terms with all of this the quickest, probably because I kind of *had* to. It took a little longer to convince the rest of my family, but it was worth it.

It was a slow process, but Michael's sleeping just got better and better as time went on. At first, I was talking about sleep on every appointment we had with Jonathan. But by the four-month visit, we didn't have to talk about it at all.

As for why I needed to train Michael for so long, but Nicholas settled into it naturally? Who knows. It goes to show you that every baby really is different. It's all the more reason not to take anything for granted, and to do what you can to give your baby good habits.

The Mom Whose First Child Slept So Little That She Felt Totally Wiped Out All the Time

KRISTEN T.

I don't drink a lot, but I think that's what it was like. It was like being drunk. All the time.

My first son, Frankie, was born three years ago, and from the beginning, he didn't give us a moment's peace. He seemed to cry constantly. If he went longer than forty-five minutes without crying, that seemed good. It was twenty-four hours a day, and the only thing that would quiet him was the bottle. So we were basically feeding him around-the-clock.

I could barely keep my eyes open most of the day. I was in sweatpants all the time and I was usually covered in spit-up. But I barely felt like getting in the shower, I was so tired. The only thing I could compare it to, the only way I could describe the sleep deprivation, that felt like I was giving people a fair impression of how I felt, was to say it was like being drunk.

Our pediatrician at the time was not much of a help. He wasn't very informative, or instructive about what we could do to make things easier, let alone at all *normal*.

A neighbor of ours is a second grade teacher, and she's always in the know when it comes to the goings-on of children and parents in our town. She recommended that we go see Jonathan Jassey; she had heard great things about him.

I told Jonathan about my experience with my son up to that point, and, almost immediately, he suspected that Frankie might have a milk protein allergy.

Then Jonathan examined him and did some tests and we found out that yes, Frankie was allergic to milk and soy. That was probably why he had been having so much difficulty and why nothing we had tried seemed to work.

Knowing Frankie had these allergies helped solve one problem; we started feeding him a hypoallergenic formula and he was now able to keep more milk down, and he became much happier in general.

But we still had a major problem. Frankie's eating and particularly sleeping habits had been horribly "off" for five weeks. Even with the milk allergies accounted for, we had our work cut out for us in undoing the "routine" that was already established.

Jonathan told us we had to start working to get Frankie on a stable, consistent schedule as soon as possible. At that point, we were grateful anytime Frankie was asleep; that's how rarely it seemed to take place. We would never dream of waking him when he was sleeping. But Jonathan taught us that we had to take that mind-set and throw it out the window; to get Frankie on a reliable schedule, we'd have to wake him if he was asleep when it was the proper time for a feeding. And getting him on a schedule was the key; it was the thing that would filter into everything else we did to take care of Frankie, and make it all easier.

We began extending the time between feedings by around fifteen minutes each day, and slowly but surely, we worked our way into a rhythm.

Finally, after a few weeks, we had Frankie consistently feeding every four hours—or at least close to that—during the day. And he was sleeping from 9 p.m. to around 3 a.m. at night, which, compared to how things had been going before we met Jonathan, was amazing.

But Jonathan reminded us that that wasn't a good schedule.

"Even if we can only get him sleeping five hours overnight, then we'll have to accept that," he said. "But we want those five hours to at least be at the right time. We want it to be after midnight, so you can get some sleep, too."

That meant we had to wake Frankie up at midnight to feed if he was sleeping. We didn't want to do that at first, but we trusted

Jonathan. Everything he had advised us to do so far had been right on the money.

"I promise you are doing a great job," Jonathan would say. "And in a few weeks, you are going to have a baby that's sleeping all the way through the night."

So we started waking Frankie for a midnight feeding. And pretty soon after that, he was going from midnight to around 6 or 7 in the morning. At around eleven weeks old, Frankie was finally sleeping through the night without interruption. And we were able to return to a semi-normal existence.

If you had told me that that would be possible only six weeks earlier, when Frankie couldn't go more than an hour without waking up and crying, and I was walking around un-showered, covered in spit-up and feeling drunk all day—I never would have believed it.

But amazingly, when our second son, Jessie, was born a couple of months ago, I had basically forgotten everything we went through with Frankie. Maybe I had been repressing it or something. Whatever the case, when Jessie came home, we didn't start sleep training him immediately. I don't know why.

Luckily, Jessie naturally had pretty good sleep habits. He automatically only needed the bottle every four hours or so, and we never felt out of control with his feedings, like we had with Frankie. The only issue was that Jessie woke up every night at around 2 or 3 a.m. When that happened, we'd give him an ounce or two of milk, and he'd go back to sleep pretty easily.

Compared to our ordeal with Frankie, we were practically happy to only have to wake up once a night for Jessie, even if it was at 2 or 3 a.m. But Jonathan said we should try to get rid of that feeding. He was always patient with us, but he always reminded us that if we didn't *want* to be waking up then, we didn't have to. But it depended on getting Jessie to not expect that 2 a.m. milk infusion.

"Just remember," Jonathan said. "They wake up if they're used to getting milk at a certain time. But if they realize they're not going to get what they want, then they're not going to wake up. If you change what his little stomach expects, it will change what his mind expects."

From then on, when Jessie would wake up in the middle of the night crying in his crib, I'd go into his room and play a "game" with him. I'd put the pacifier in his mouth, and then lie down next to the crib, catching whatever "z's" I could. It was a game, because after some time sucking on it, Jessie would inevitably spit the pacifier out of his mouth, I'd hear it bounce against the crib, and I'd get up and put it back in.

Each night, I was determined to play the game at least fifteen minutes longer than the previous night. If he was still crying at that point, I'd give him a little milk so we could both go back to sleep. Eventually our game could last as long as an hour and a half, which at 3 in the morning could be excruciating. But I kept reminding myself of what Jonathan always said:

"I promise you are doing a great job. And in a few weeks, you are going to have a baby that's sleeping all the way through the night."

Sure enough, after several days, Jessie stopped crying in the middle of the night, and slept from midnight until 6 a.m. (Or maybe he was waking up, and self-soothing. Either way, he was doing well, and he wasn't waking *us* up.) At 6 a.m., Jessie only wanted an ounce of two of milk anyway, so after a few more mornings of giving him the pacifier at that point, we were able to eliminate that feeding. At seven and a half weeks, Jessie was now sleeping from midnight to 8:30 a.m. Then we were even able to eliminate the midnight feeding, and he'd go from 10 p.m. to 8:30 a.m.

When it starts working, it's simply magical. Yes, it's tough at first, but pretty soon you're getting five hours a night, then the next thing you know, you're getting eight hours and then twelve hours. I recommend the Jassey Way to all new moms I know. A lot of them say it sounds crazy, but I just tell them what Jonathan always told me.

"If you want your baby to sleep through the night," I say. "This is the only way it's going to happen."

Some moms come back to me and say, "I tried it, but it didn't work."

With respect to them, I would guess that they give up trying to get to a full three or four hours between feedings, and that they cave in after two hours or so if their baby cries. I've been there. It's tough!

But it's worth it.

The Dad Who Became a Baby Sleep Master

ANDREW H.

My wife, Eliza, and I met the Jasseys when we had our first daughter, Sydney, and we fell in love with them instantly. We never thought of going anywhere else after that. They seemed to embody the new, young—I almost want to say hip—way of doing things, compared to other doctors we had seen. The Jasseys were forward-thinking. To me, they always seemed to be about so much more than medicine. It was about the feeding and the sleeping and the happiness of everyone—not just the health of everyone.

I remember exactly what Jonathan said to us on the first visit.

He looked right at us and, referring to Sydney, said, "Are you interested in getting her to sleep through the night?" As if anyone would ever say "no" to that question. We said, "Yes, of course."

Then we did exactly what he told us to sleep train the baby and it worked perfectly with almost no extra thought about it.

We were steadfast about not giving Sydney the bottle when she was crying if it wasn't time to feed her, because we had watched a few other people we knew make that mistake. We went into having kids knowing not to do a couple of things and that was on the list. I think that it was very important to our success.

We have a one-year-old named Jordan now, as well; we used the Jasseys' method with her, too. Fortunately, neither daughter put us to the test too much at night. I never had to sit and listen to either of them cry at night for an hour and a half, and worry about not giving up and giving them the bottle.

My wife breast-fed our daughters, so at the hospital, they had her feeding every two hours right away.

Then Dr. Jassey said that he wanted us to try to get that to three hours between feedings, and when we reached that, at the next appointment he said he wanted us to try to go for four hours. Then at the next appointment, he had us get rid of the middle of the night feeding. It all pretty much fell into place.

But it's not that there weren't a lot of times when it didn't seem to be going 100 percent perfectly, when questions came up, and we didn't know exactly what to do.

For instance, the baby would be due for a bottle at three hours, but she'd be sleeping, and it would be the middle of the day.

Should we wake her up and give her that bottle exactly at three hours because if we don't, then she might go too long and screw up the rest of the schedule? What effect will it have on the rest of the day and evening? Will we have to recalculate everything?

Then we'd ask Dr Jassey and he said not to wake her up.

"Let it go," he would say. "See how long she'll give you."

It wasn't an exact science.

In the beginning, the schedule changes over and over again because you keep making it a little bit further during the night.

I would memorize the spreads. I remember saying to my wife, "We're on the one, five, nine now," referring to the feeding schedule: one o'clock, five o'clock and nine o'clock.

But the next day, it could be a "two, six, ten" kind of thing.

It goes back and forth until eventually you've taken away that night feeding completely, and she sleeps through the night.

At one point, there really is a miraculous moment like that. There's no other way to describe it. It didn't all happen exactly according to the math.

One day you wake up in the morning and look at your wife and say, "Wow, she just slept from one o'clock in the morning to six a.m.! That's five hours; it's the biggest spread we've ever had." Then that turns into six hours, then seven hours, and goes on like that. You're constantly pushing the numbers ahead.

The baby's feeding schedule is never going to resemble a normal adult's schedule of three meals a day—until she's a toddler. So you can't think of it as breakfast, lunch and dinner and an overnight feeding.

While she's still a baby, you have to think of it as an every-three-hour thing that turns into an every-four-hour thing, that turns into an every-five-hour thing, until it does become three or four meals during the day with a long overnight stretch between meals.

Except that while you let them go as long as possible overnight, during the day you wouldn't let them go longer than four hours between feedings.

I think the reason that the Jasseys' technique doesn't work for some parents is that it's so easy to think a kid is hungry when she actually isn't. You think she needs the food because she's crying, but she doesn't. You have to be able to resist that; you have to be able to say "no."

Another big mistake is getting too wrapped up in how the feeding schedule is going to affect your *own* schedule. Some people don't want to reorient their life to fit the baby being fed at this or that particular time. You have to make that little sacrifice in the beginning for it to work in the long run.

My three-year-old still sleeps ten to twelve hours a night. She doesn't wake up at the crack of dawn and come running into our bedroom to wake us up, as the kids of some of our friends do. She wakes up between 7 or 8 in the morning and contents herself until I go in there.

There have been times where *I've* had to wake up both my daughters in the morning, because I had to go to work and I wanted to say good-bye.

The Mom Who Traded Fifteen Minutes for Eight Hours

JESSICA S.

I remember taking my daughter Skylar to Dr. Lewis Jassey for her two- or three-week-old appointment, and he told me I could get her sleeping through the night if I followed a few tips from him.

Skylar had been used to feeding every three hours, and Lewis suggested that we try to push each feeding back by fifteen minutes.

"If you start this today," he said, "you're going to get five or six hours of sleep tonight."

I started as soon as we got home that day; I thought maybe it would start working in a day or two. But that same night she went from waking up every two hours to getting five hours of sleep.

It can be hard to do, because sometimes you've got a screaming baby on your hands, and the last thing you want to do is hear your child scream or cry like that.

"When she's crying, she's not starving to death, and she's not in pain," Dr. Jassey would tell me. "It's okay for her to cry." That's what I would tell myself when I'd be rocking her to sleep instead of feeding her.

Now she's two months old, and she sleeps eight hours every single night.

I tell people that, and their jaws drop open.

I know Dr. Jassey recommends four hours between feedings, and I never let Skylar go longer than that, but ever since we went from three hours to just 3:15 between feedings, it helped her sleep overnight. She still seems to want to feed at three hours sometimes—she'll start crying—but as long as I wait at least another fifteen minutes, she'll give me that eight-hour stretch overnight.

On the other hand, it's very hard for my husband to hear her cry, and sometimes he'll feed her before that 3:15 mark. When that happens, she doesn't sleep through the night.

I don't know what it is about those fifteen minutes for her, or how it works, but it's amazing. Maybe it's just a matter of her not expecting the bottle just because she's crying.

Sometimes a baby is screaming her head off, and it can be very difficult to not feed her. That bottle's right there, and you know you can stick it in her mouth and have a quiet baby. But if you can get past that reflex, you're golden.

My mother comes over all the time and when the baby's crying, she'll say, "Just feed her."

But I'm the one who's going to be kept up at night, not her.

The Mom Who Was So Successful She Had to Hide It

MEREDITH W.

Dr. Jon and I are very close friends, and my first son, Zachary, was Jonathan's first official patient after he completed his training. When Jon told us about this method of sleep training, I didn't know anything else about baby sleep. "Whatever Jon says," I thought, "I'll do."

Our parents had a tough time with it. They were against waiting four hours between feedings. Their generation learned a completely different way of approaching all of this.

But Zachary was sleeping straight through the night by the time he was ten days old. From eleven o'clock at night until seven o'clock in the morning.

People resented me for how successful it was. Friends of mine, even. I became afraid to tell people that my husband and I were getting eight to nine hours of sleep with a newborn baby in the house. The first question people usually ask you after you have a baby is "Are you sleeping?" I would have to bite my tongue. I'd say something like, "Yeah, we're sleeping. We're getting by." But the truth was, he was sleeping for eight hours straight without a problem.

It really worked to a T. And we were able to do it gradually, which was great. The first night, he went about four and a half hours overnight. Then we just extended it each night, until he was going eight hours. It was textbook.

Zach had bad reflux and was on medication for it, but the method still worked perfectly. It was unbelievable.

The only issue was that it set the bar so high for my second son, Brandon. It took him about ten weeks to sleep through the night. But it was never a food issue with him. It was more like he'd wake up at two or three in the morning and want to play and hang out. He never woke up crying from hunger. The method totally satisfied his stomach for a twenty-four-hour period.

And the bottom line is that both kids were sleeping for eight hours before they were three months old.

The Second-Time Mom Who Wasn't Going to Make That Mistake Again

DANIELLE S.

With my first child, I was a little bit soft. I wasn't tough enough to follow what Dr. Lewis was recommending. I couldn't stand to hear the baby crying, so it was hard to train him. And he'd wake up in the middle of the night at least three times. At twelve, two and four. When he got a little older, it became two times a night. But he's three years old now, and he still wakes up in the middle of the night!

When he was waking up three times every night, I wasn't sleeping very much at all. It was very difficult. So with my second child, I thought, "We have to do something different."

This time I followed the method, and he was sleeping at one month. I'd give him an extra ounce of milk with the last feeding, and when he woke up the first night, I let him cry for fifteen minutes before feeding him. Then the next night, I let him go thirty minutes. He'd cry, but I knew it was okay. When my first child would cry, I'd run to him after only two minutes. This time I knew I had to do it differently. I'd make him comfortable, but I wouldn't feed him.

Every night, we went fifteen minutes longer. And then after about a week, he started sleeping through the night. I think it clicked with him that if he woke up and cried, he wasn't going to get the bottle. So he stopped.

I have a good friend who just had twins, and I told her about the Jassey Way, and it's working for her. They're waking up once a night now, instead of two times. As a first-time mom, you don't want to hear them cry at all. But she has two newborns, so it would be even tougher for her to not get sleep. Twins are so much work.

I tell everyone about it now. It's nice to be able to control the baby's sleep. A lot of people don't know it, but there's a way to do it. I'm glad we did.

But it's not just for us. When the baby gets a good night's sleep, he's less cranky the next day. It's good for everyone.

If I could go back in time, I'd do it with my first child, too. It's not as hard as you think it's going to be.

CHAPTER TEN

Glossary of Terms

The following words and phrases are by no means "must know" terms. Heck, most of them aren't even medical terms!

We wanted to include this list because these words and this "language" illustrate our perspective on baby care. You might say this glossary is a good summary of *our* big-picture view of things.

We hope these terms resonate with you, almost like little baby care "mantras," and that they help guide you in caring for your little one.

24-hour drive-thru—A fast-food restaurant that stays open all night, so you can drive over to it and pick up late-night greasy food when you have that particular craving. Not what you need to be for your infant.

China—The farthest location patients of ours have moved to and still come back for checkups. (One dad's job was relocated there.

The family always gets in touch when they come back to New York.)

Chronic infections—What sleep-deprived children can get due to compromised immune systems.

Colic—An empty term used to refer to a "cranky" baby when a deeper cause is not known.

Creature of habit—What every human is (including babies).

Cry it out method—Not something the Jassey Way advocates. Instead, we recommend rocking, singing, reading and otherwise engaging with your baby to calm her in the middle of the night—without resorting to an unnecessary feeding.

Dream feed—The last bottle of the night, if the baby is basically only half-awake.

Eggshells—What people tend to walk on nowadays when discussing babies, in lieu of speaking the plain truth.

Enabling—Something that can be all too inadvertently successful with babies. Being creatures of habit, babies are all too easily influenced. We'd be well advised to enable their healthy, constructive behavior and habits—as opposed to reinforcing behavior that is consistently inconsistent and all too potentially harmful.

Front end—The last feeding before bed.

Full tank of gas—What you want a newborn to have going into a night's sleep; a result of a turkey feeding (the larger-than-normal final feeding of the night, which, like a Thanksgiving feast, will put your newborn to sleep).

Golden Rule—The longer a baby goes between feedings, the longer she'll be able to sleep.

Grazing—Eating a little bit at a time, countless times per day. *Not* what you want your baby to be doing—unless you want to be feeding your baby 24/7 and not sleeping at all yourself.

Head/stomach—Two organs that are directly linked in a baby's body, and can be conditioned accordingly to achieve meaningful sleep.

Higher expectations—What we have for a baby's ability to sleep through the night.

Human pacifier—What some parents make themselves, rather than letting their babies learn how to self-soothe.

Jassey Way—A commonsense method for getting a newborn to sleep for at least seven hours a night.

Jet lag—The residual effect for a newborn of one bad night's sleep on the next day, and on the next night's sleep.

Jiminy Cricket—A good pediatrician should serve as the conscience of parents, helping them to avoid giving in to quick, unproductive fixes for issues their children have.

Jonathan's Stand—The two-week period during and after Superstorm Sandy when Jonathan didn't veer from his infant daughter's feeding schedule, even though there was no power in the house, there was pandemonium all around, and letting the child nurse a bottle all day long would have solved a lot of other, non-baby issues.

Lightbulb—Something that you can't expect to magically appear above a baby's head, as baby realizes when and how long to be asleep for.

Marcus Welby, MD—The kind of whole-family, house-call type of doctor we aspire to be.

Mom's antibodies—What a newborn's immune system consists of up to the first six months of life; it's fragile, and extra-susceptible to being compromised by sleep-deprivation.

Nocturnal creature—What a baby should not be.

On-demand channel—What a parent need not be for a newborn.

One long stretch/the DiMaggio—The at least seven hours of sleep almost every baby is capable of at night.

Pacifier—A baby-quieting accessory sometimes called a binky. A pacifier is also what your baby should not view feeding as.

Pediatrics—A branch of medicine that, contrary to popular belief, deals not only with the medical care of infants, children and adolescents, but with whole families, with a focus on the children.

Physical and mental exhaustion—What a sleepless baby can engender in a couple.

Puppy—An animal not as smart as a newborn, and yet thought of as more trainable.

Purgatory—Where exhausted parents can find themselves. Some say it's a land without sleep training.

Reflux—A common cause of baby displeasure and crying.

Ripple effect—The deleterious effect that a sleepless baby can have on the rest of the family.

Rocket science—What the Jassey Way is not.

Self-soothing—An essential life skill that is best acquired as soon as possible. Settling into sleep is an excellent way for babies to learn to self-soothe.

Sex drive—What a sleepless baby can destroy in a couple.

Short-term solution—A harsh but fair word for feeding a baby in the middle of the night only because of crying.

Simple math—What the Jassey Way is.

Stretch out—To expand the amount of sleep an infant gets at night, via the Jassey Way.

Teething—A common cause of baby displeasure and crying temperament.

ACKNOWLEDGMENTS

DR. LEWIS JASSEY

I want to thank my wife, Orna, for encouraging me to pursue this dream of sharing this brainchild with the world. You have the greatest job in the world and do it so beautifully: cultivating the minds and values of our two wonderful daughters. They couldn't possibly be where they are today without you. You are my sounding board, you are my backbone and you are my Jiminy Cricket. And I hope this experience will allow me to find a new appreciation for how books are like oxygen to you. I love you much too much.

To my thirteen-year-old daughter, Julia: I want to thank you for blessing me with the gift of watching you grow up. Your heart is of golden fibers, your soul is of celestial fabric and your writing is like that of a prodigy. I hope when I grow up, I can be half as talented as you. The world will most certainly know who you are someday. And your first book will be more of a success than this one, I have no doubt.

To my eight-year-old daughter, Mya, I want to thank you, too, for providing me with the treasure of vicariously living through you. Your determination is unbending, your common sense and sense of humor are both decades above your chronological age, and your mathematical wizardry is fascinating and seamless. You will always have an impossibly big heart. Keep the dream of being the president . . . and opening up that donut shop in the White House!

I want to thank my brothers, Adam and Jonathan, for being so tight with me growing up. I'm so thankful we were there for each other during some real tough times. I'm so proud of both of you. I still have to pinch myself from time to time when I think that Jonathan and I get to live out a lifelong dream of working together. Love you, bros!

I want to give a special acknowledgment to my stepfather, Bob. You have been there for my brothers and me so many times over the years, including some very difficult times. But more than that, you were there for our mom. When you came into her life, you simply put a smile on her face, a smile that was long overdue. And that smile has never left her. On behalf of my brothers and me, I thank you so much for that. You never tried to be a father, only a friend. And you've been a rather good one.

There were so many teachers along the way that truly made a difference. Mrs. Bailin, Mrs. Polan, Mr. Koenig, Mr. Shaldone, Dr. Boxer, Dr. Balbi, and Dr. Miller were the difference makers.

I want to thank all the wonderful staff I have had with me at Bellmore Merrick Pediatrics and Adolescent Medicine over the years. They say you can't choose your family, but see, here at my office, I have. You incredible people have helped genuinely care for all the unbelievable families that I have been blessed to have been a part of. So many of these success stories couldn't have been pulled off without all of you.

And to all those amazing families, thank you as well, for allowing me into your lives. It's a real privilege to be able to care for someone's child, and one that I will never take for granted. So many special memories in that pediatric office!

I also want to thank Byrd Leavell for believing in a dream of the Jassey brothers, and Colby Brin for providing such an enjoyable experience while working with him.

Lastly, I'd like to thank Chuck D for the lesson of the power of the spoken word, and George Brett, for the lesson in passion when thrown out of the Pine Tar Game.

I thank G-d for you all, and for giving me the opportunity to wake up every single day, drive to work and love what I'm doing with my life.

DR. JONATHAN JASSEY

I want to thank my loving and beautiful wife, Suzanne, for her support and belief in me. Thank you for being there for me through the years. You could've walked away when I was in medical school and didn't always have the time for you because of studying, but you stuck it out, and look at the beautiful family we have made. You are always in my corner and I couldn't be happier waking up next to my soul mate every day of my life.

And my three beautiful kids, Charli, Camryn and Harper, for letting me practice what I preach. You made my talks to patients that much easier since I could give them examples of what each of you did as babies. You girls are the best accomplishment of my life. The time watching you grow is going by way too fast. I wish I could press pause for a little while. Life comes sort of full circle; I was one of three boys, and now I have three girls. I hope you will always remain as close as I have with my brothers. I love you all with everything that I am.

My mom, Carla, and stepfather, Bob, as well as my late father, for helping shape me into the compassionate doctor that I am. My mom always pushed me in my academics so I could be where I am today. If it weren't for her, who knows where I would be. Thanks, Mom, for always taking care of me and nurturing me in so many ways. My stepfather has been like a second father to me, and an even better friend. Thanks, Bob, for helping raise me, just when you thought you were done raising kids!

My brothers, Lewis and Adam, for being like father figures to me growing up, and to Lewis, for mentoring me as I followed in his footsteps. We've been through a lot together and I couldn't have asked for better brothers. The memories we've shared through sports, wrestling, food and everything else will last a lifetime.

Colby Brin, for all his help.

Byrd Leavell and Marian Lizzi, our literary agent and editor at Perigee, respectively, who helped us to spread the word to the masses.

To Bryan Calka, my closest friend, who always was there for my family through the years and helped connect me to Byrd to make this all happen.

To the rest of my friends and family, thank you for all you do. You all mean so much to me.

To the wonderful doctors and nursing staff at Winthrop University Hospital who taught me so much and guided me in the journey of becoming a pediatrician. You helped mold me into the doctor I am today.

And to all the great staff at Bellmore Merrick Pediatrics and Adolescent Medicine for making this practice continuously grow and for being great colleagues and friends. You guys are awesome!

RESOURCES

BOOKS

Ezzo, Gary, and Robert Bucknam. *On Becoming Baby Wise: Giving Your Infant the Gift of Nighttime Sleep.* Louisiana, MO: Parent-Wise Solutions, 2006.

Pantley, Elizabeth. *The No-Cry Sleep Solution: Gentle Ways to Help Your Baby Sleep Through the Night.* Chicago: Contemporary, 2002.

Sears, William. *The Baby Sleep Book: The Complete Guide to a Good Night's Rest for the Whole Family.* New York: Little, Brown, 2005.

Waldburger, Jennifer, and Jill Spivack. *The Sleepeasy Solution: The Exhausted Parent's Guide to Getting Your Child to Sleep—from Birth to Age Five.* Deerfield Beach, FL: Health Communications, 2007.

JOURNAL ARTICLES

Henderson, J. M., K. G. France, J. L. Owens, and N. M. Blampied. "Sleeping Through the Night: The Consolidation of Self-Regulated Sleep Across the First Year of Life." *Pediatrics* 126, no. 5 (November 2010): e1081–1087. ncbi.nlm.nih.gov/pubmed/20974775.

INTRODUCTION: THE NEWBORN SLEEP PROBLEM

1 Henderson, J. M., K. G. France, J. L. Owens, and N. M. Blampied. "Sleeping Through the Night: The Consolidation of Self-Regulated Sleep Across the First Year of Life," *Pediatrics* 126, no. 5 (November 2010): e1081–1087. ncbi.nlm.nih.gov/pubmed/20974775.

CHAPTER 3: THE CRYING GAME

1 "Colic and Crying." Medline Plus. August 2, 2011. nlm.nih.gov/medline plus/ency/article/000978.htm.

2 "Milk Allergy in Infants." KidsHealth, October 2011. kidshealth.org /parent/medical/allergies/milk_allergy.html.

CHAPTER 4: WHAT'S THE BIG DEAL ABOUT ALL THIS ANYWAY?

1 Jones, Jeffrey M. "In U.S., 40% Get Less Than Recommended Amount of Sleep." Gallup: Well-Being, December 19, 2013. gallup.com/poll/166553 /less-recommended-amount-sleep.aspx?utm_source=alert&utm_medium =email&utm_campaign=syndication&utm_content=morelink&utm _term=USA%20-%20Well-Being.

2 Schocker, Lauren. "Here's a Horrifying Picture of What Sleep Loss Will Do to You." *Huffington Post*, January 8, 2014. huffingtonpost.com/2014 /01/08/sleep-deprivation_n_4557142.html?utm_hp_ref=mostpopular.

CHAPTER 5: OF BREAST AND BOTTLE

1 "Breastfeeding vs. Formula Feeding." KidsHealth, January 2012. kids health.org/parent/growth/feeding/breast_bottle_feeding.html.

2 Ip, Stanley, Mei Chung, Gowri Raman, et al. "Breastfeeding and Maternal and Infant Health Outcomes in Developed Countries." *Evidence Reports/Technology Assessments* 153 (April 2007). ncbi.nlm.nih.gov/books /NBK38337.

3 "The Scientific Benefits of Breastfeeding." *PhD in Parenting,* May 14, 2009. phdinparenting.com/blog/2009/5/14/the-scientific-benefits-of-breast feeding.html.

4 Ibid.

CHAPTER 7: LET'S EAT

1 Iannelli, Vincent. "Baby Food Stages and Steps." About.com Pediatrics. December 4, 2004, pediatrics.about.com/od/weeklyquestion/a/04_baby _food.htm.

CHAPTER 8: COMMON QUESTIONS, SAMPLE SCHEDULES AND WELL BABY EXAMS

1 "Safe to Sleep." Public Education Campaign. December 19, 2013. nichd .nih.gov/sts/Pages/default.aspx.